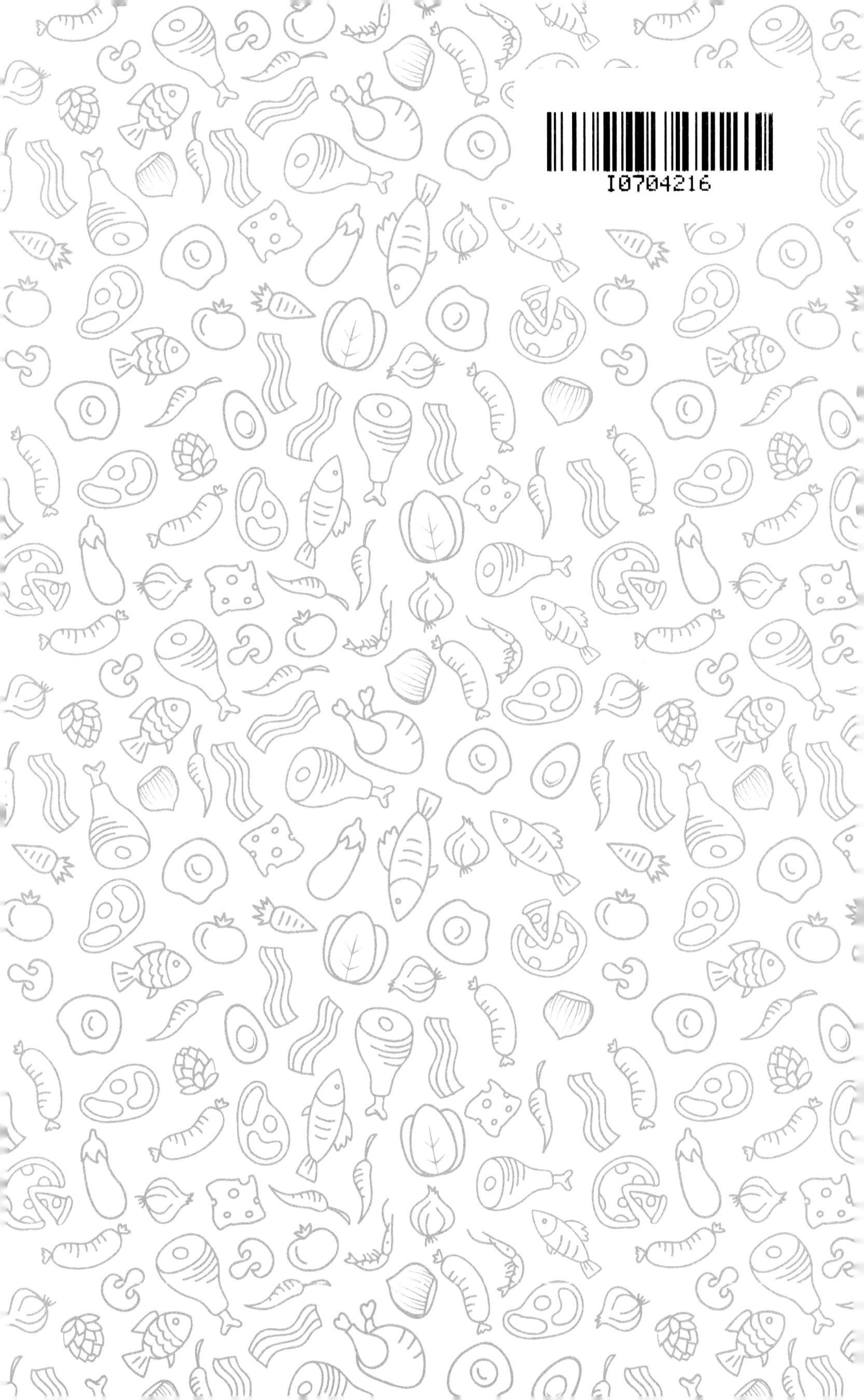
I0704216

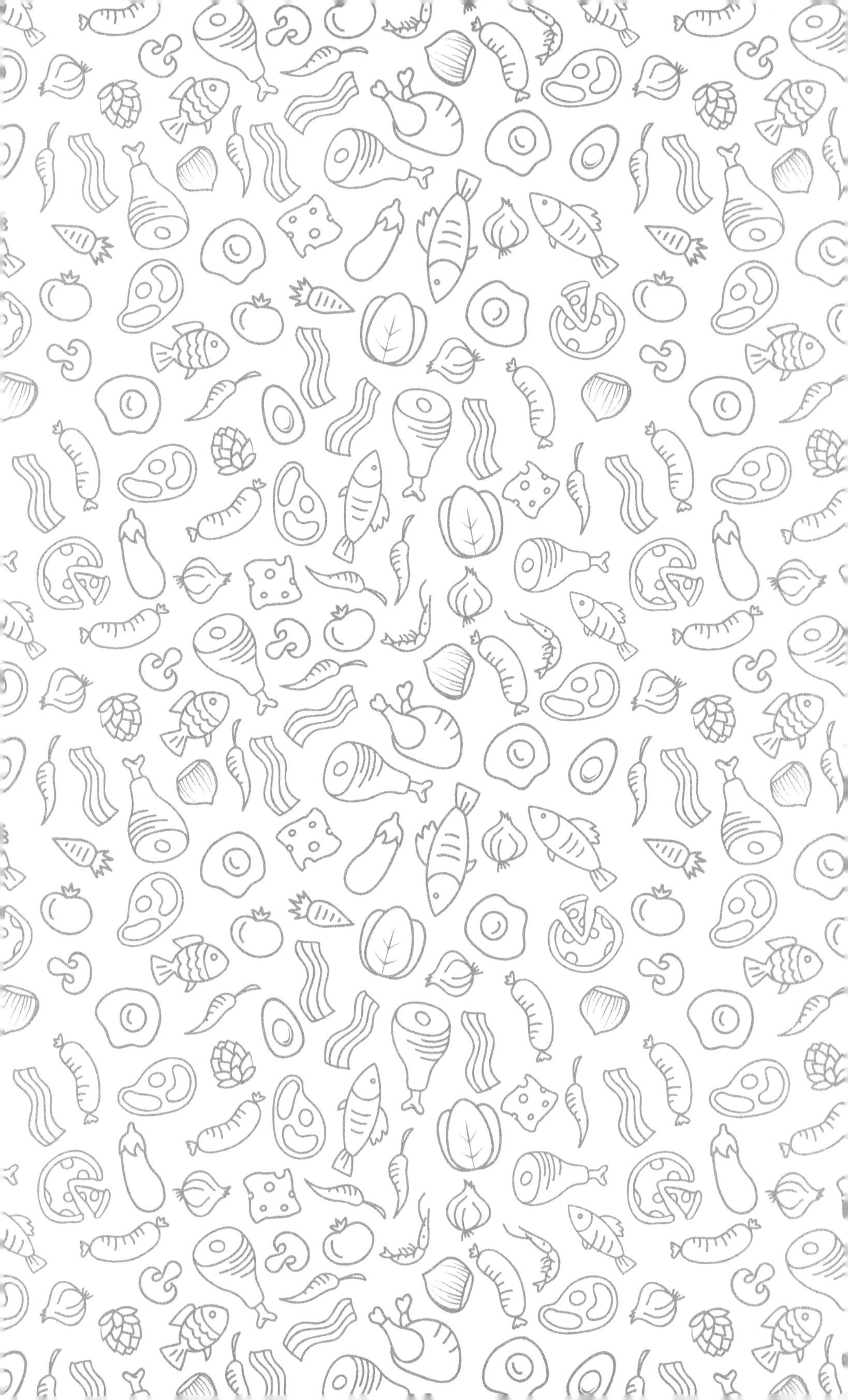

TJAŠA VRHOVNIK & GAŠPER GROM

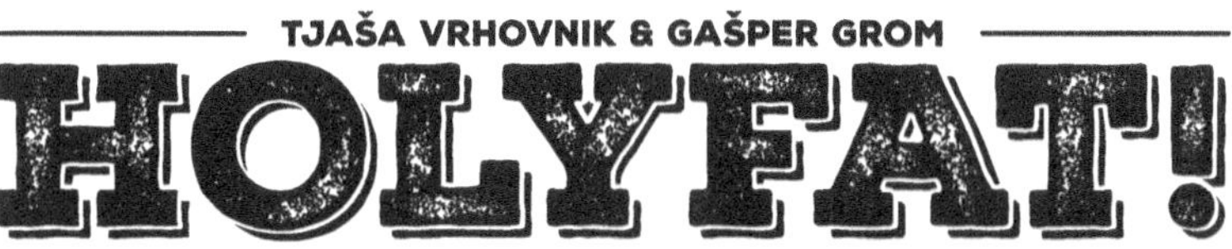

HOLYFAT!

How DIETARY FATS *can help you* LOSE WEIGHT & FEEL GOOD

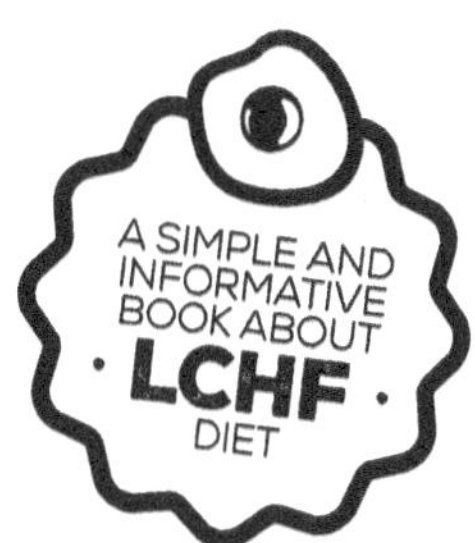

HOLY FAT!
How dietary fats can help you lose weight and feel good
Tjaša Vrhovnik and Gašper Grom

First published with the title "Bemumast! Z uživanjem maščob do vitkosti in dobrega počutja", Slovenija 2016

Published by: **Keto Love Ltd., UK**
Book design and photography: **Tjaša Vrhovnik**
Translation: **Simon Bolčević, PSD d. o. o.**
Editing: **Christian Green**
Revision: **Beth Zupec-Kania**

The book Holy Fat! is an informative book describing the LCHF (low carb high fat) diet, or the ketogenic diet. It contains a collection of all currently available information regarding this diet, originating directly from scientific literature, and in some parts from the personal experience of Gašper Grom, a LCHF nutritionist. The book does not wish to, and can't replace, a consultation with a physician or a specialist.

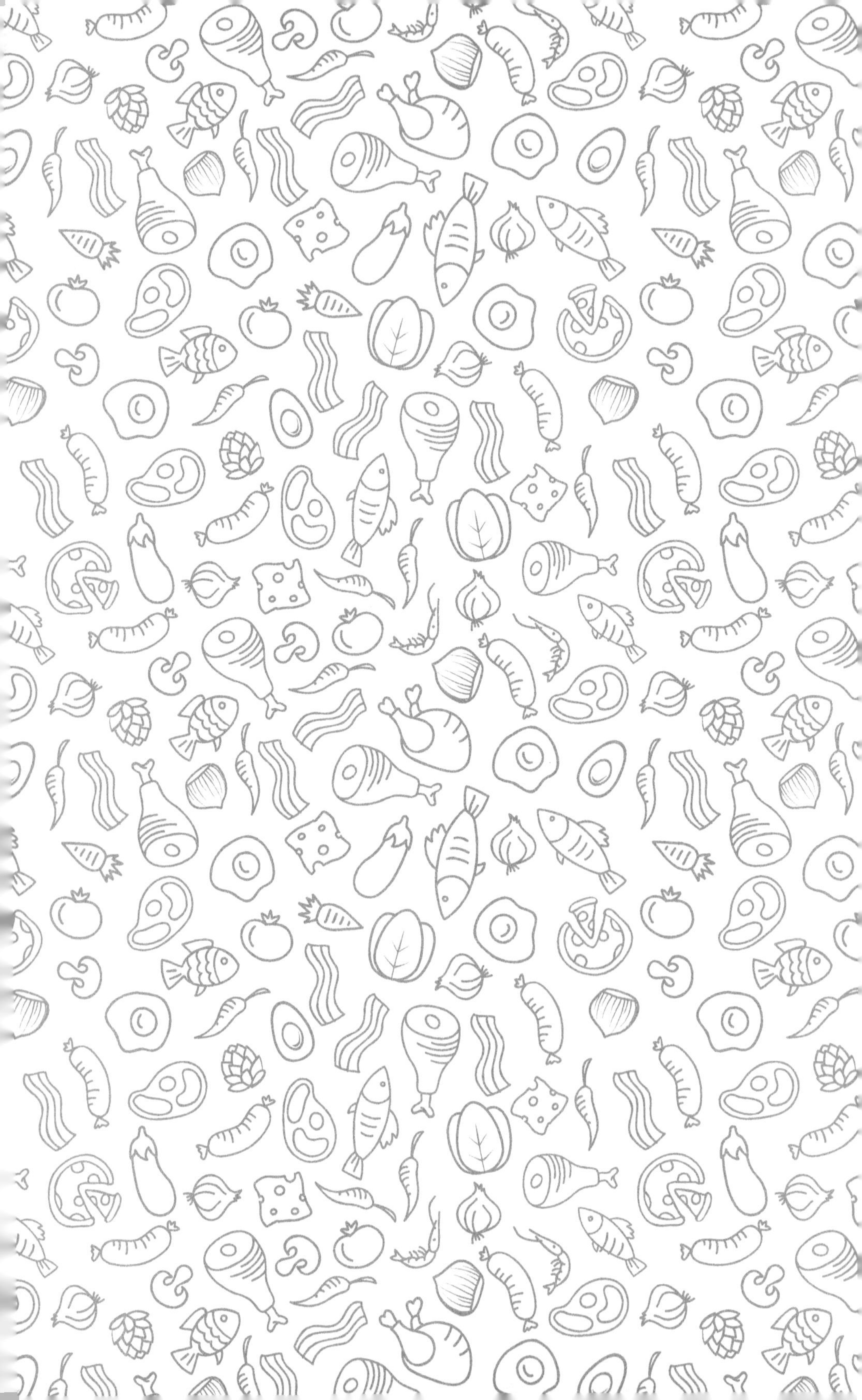

CONTENTS

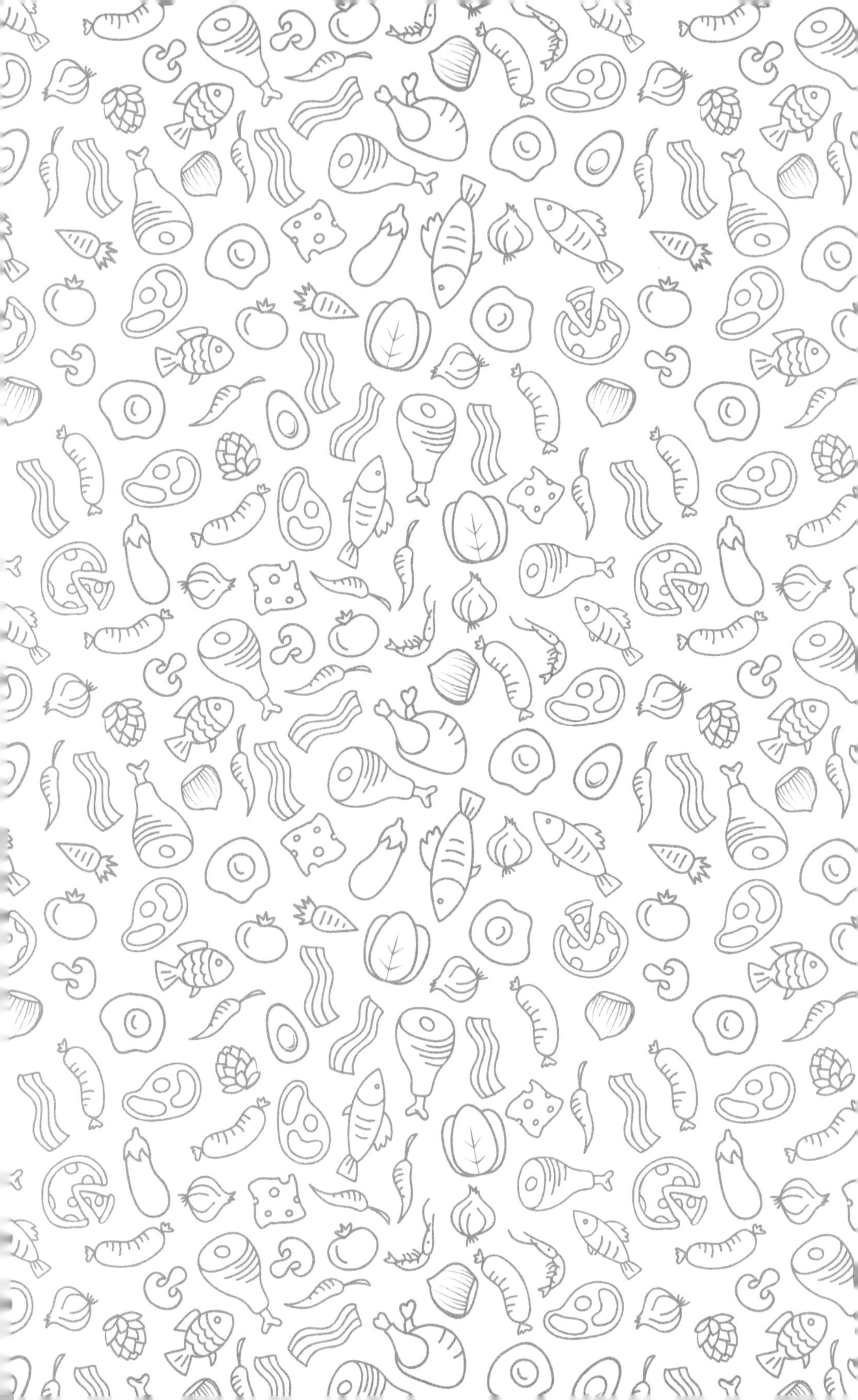

10 BENEFITS OF THE LCHF DIET

1. The end of constantly feeling hungry and the end of hunger itself.

2. Craving desserts, pizzas and other carbohydrate rich foods becomes just an unpleasant memory.

3. Fewer meals required; often even three meals a day prove to be too much.

4. A reduced waist circumference and subsequently less belly fat, which is not only aesthetically unpleasing, but can lead to dangerous inflammation that presents grounds for the development of serious disease.

5. A distinct improvement of the lipid levels in blood (cholesterol and triglycerides). Doctors will be astonished!

6. Stabilized blood sugar and lower levels of insulin. If you have diabetes and take prescribed medication, it is possible that it can be reduced or eliminated.

7. Lower blood pressure.

8. Improved mental capacity and better focus.

9. An end to constantly feeling unwell, fatigued or lacking in energy.

10. A diverse diet that looks appetizing and appealing.

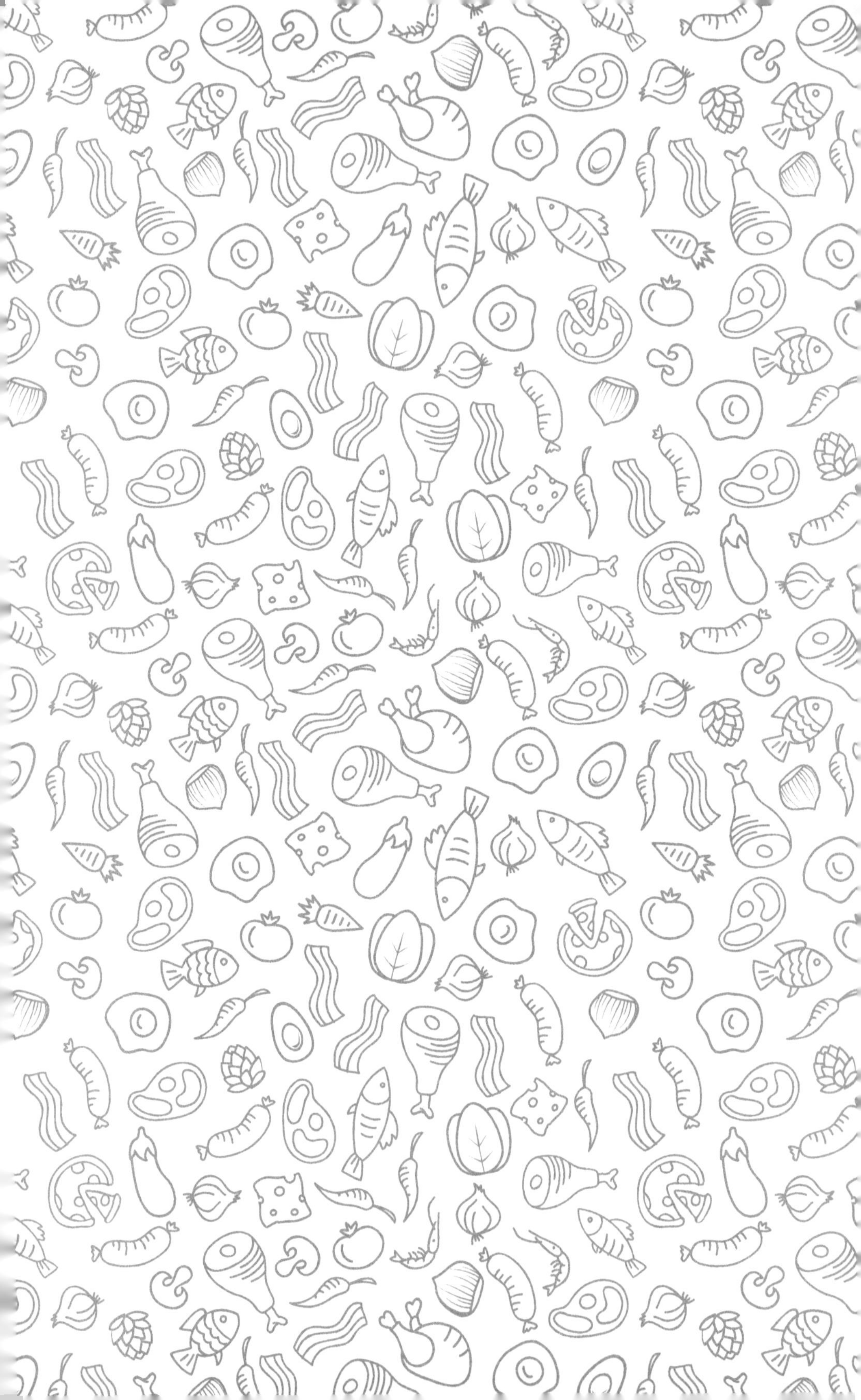

INTRODUCTION

The book you are holding in your hands is primarily intended for individuals who wish to change the composition of their body. Informally, this is called dieting, but just as all pizzas don't taste great, not all forms of weight loss are good for you. You can lose weight with the excessive use of laxatives or by not eating anything for a week. While the latter may not be easy, it is achievable. It is also possible to lose weight by eating nothing but cabbage soup for long periods of time - this option is also less expensive than using laxatives. There's an infinite amount of ways to lose weight, but so is stupidity most probably – as Albert Einstein once stated: there are only two things which are infinite, the universe and human stupidity, and he wasn't sure about the former.

The issues with these methods is the fact that you do not get rid of what you carry in excess; body fat deposits. I'm sure you understand that by cutting off your own leg you will weigh less – and you're smart enough not to use this approach; without that leg your life wouldn't be the same as it was with both. This principle can be applied when dieting. You don't want to be dehydrated, you don't want to flush out your gut flora, you don't want to lose musculoskeletal tissue and you definitely don't want to suffer by eating that nasty cabbage soup. In the same fashion, you wouldn't chop your leg off just because of a number on a scale.

We can therefore conclude that you wish to change your body's composition by lowering the amount of body fat, maintaining a healthy gut and musculoskeletal system and managing to do so with as little sacrifice, suffering and cabbage soup as possible.

Many of you have picked this book up because you have seen a friend of yours transformed from a fatty into someone with a body like the models on the front pages of fitness magazines. Others of you are reading this because you have tried and failed every single time in attempting to transform from a fatty into someone with a more acceptable and pleasing body.

Let us ruin your excitement straight away by stating that a low-carbohydrate, high-fat intake, as well as a ketogenic diet *won't* work. At least not on their own.

A person can function well if their diet is appropriate. This person, of course, is you. All of you who want to wear an outfit three sizes smaller, and those of you, who are ready for a different life, because you have finally realized what you've been doing up until this moment in regards to your diet and health has been simply atrocious.

Maybe a doctor warned you that you are at an increased risk of metabolic syndrome (a combination of belly fat, high levels of triglycerides, high blood pressure, symptoms of type 2 diabetes and low levels of HDL cholesterol), or maybe you were recommended a fat rich diet as part of your therapy in dealing with an autoimmune disease.

There is no doubt that a lot of you are sportsmen, athletes and active individuals who seek precise, minute solutions and pay extreme attention to every pound of body weight you carry. Although you have learned a lot and gained experience with a disciplined diet, you have become stuck in a rut that does not fulfill your expectations. This book is meant for you too.

This may well be the best book for the situation you're in. It may also be one of the very few books out there that doesn't promise miracles and shortcuts. You won't find sensational promises that will later leave you disappointed.

The Holy Fat! book will guide you towards reaching the goals you set for yourself and will genuinely and without any bovine feces, take you through the obstacles you will face on your journey.

Three Disclaimers for You, Precious Readers

The book is not a substitute for any kind of therapy and as such isn't meant to discourage readers from seeking medical assistance when dealing with acute or chronic medical conditions. Dietary measures described in this book CAN be fully beneficial, nevertheless we suggest consulting a doctor or two before making drastic changes to your diet, especially if you suffer from any medical conditions.

Although this book tends to expose dietary delusions of a systematic nature, which lead many people into following particular dietary routines, possibly based on false and inaccurate claims, some readers might begin to feel responsible for their issues with excess body weight. We wish to emphasize that yes, you are the one eating inappropriately, but other factors such as society, dietary recommendations and sensationalism, mostly based on tales, make matters worse. The same can be said about the dietary approaches presented in this book and this point needs to be stressed: knowledge of the complex processes of various aspects of the human metabolism is never fully irrefutable and is subject to constant critical evaluation. Even if you know someone who consumes a lot of fat and very little carbohydrates and they have, since practicing this type of diet, managed to cure themselves of an autoimmune disease, the two things may not be in any way related. It could very well be so, but not necessarily. For instance, the co-author follows the diet by consuming a very small amount of carbohydrates along with a high fat intake, yet her autoimmune disease condition hasn't improved.

The third disclaimer is intended for a special kind of people, who will no doubt reach out for this book when seeking solutions for their specific issues. We are referring to everyone with an overly emotional relationship to food, i.e. people who use food to regulate their most likely negative emotions. It is possible that a change in your intake ratio of macronutrients will prove to be beneficial for you in many ways, but it's worth considering that the way you manipulate the quantity and structure of the food you consume is simply the result of an emotional problem. Fortunately help also exists for these situations, and we urge you to seek it – it might turn out that once you solve your emotional issues, the dietary problems and consequences of it felt by your body will suddenly seem completely negligible.

None of the Diets Work – Tested! Why Should This One?

Many of you claim to have tried out all existing diets out there and none of them worked and we believe you. Although you haven't tried all of them, the bad experience from the ones you have tried made you feel as though none of them ever work. The food combining diet, 90-day diet, Mediterranean diet, cabbage soup diet, low sodium diet, yogurt diet, egg diet, lemon diet, melon diet, pineapple diet, bread stick diet, chemical breakdown diet, protein diet, salad diet, blood type diet, vegetarian diet, vegan diet, macrobiotic diet, raw food diet – all of these diets have been tested and showed no results. You've stuffed yourself with goji berries, grapefruit, spirulina, broccoli, cabbage soup (mhm), chili, you guzzled apple cider vinegar, green tea, black tea, white tea, red tea, herbal weight loss concoctions, sugar-free energy drinks, you slept in the cold, showered with ice cold water, showered with boiling hot water, you have wrapped yourself in plastic clothing, used electric stimulants and tested all kinds of commercial preparations and magical elixirs in vain.

In this day and age we hardly have enough time and knowledge to competently maneuver through all of the promises of these self-proclaimed experts, dieting magicians and greedy nutritionists, who only guarantee results if you use their XY products. Then there's the internet, TV, newspaper articles, wacky spiritualists who rob you blind for performing simple rotations of the torso and correcting your breathing, foot massages and concoctions made out of South American truffles, originally consumed by the indigenous tribes as they didn't have McDonald's at their disposal, and so on.

What do all of these things have in common?

Science.

Or nicely put: the lack of a scientific basis.

Science can be wrong. The reason we did not state that science "can unfortunately be wrong" is the fact that we consider this to be the advantage of science. Science is not a religion and in science there are no dogmas and irrefutable facts. As the British comedian John Cleese once stated, science is a method of investigation. It is NOT a belief system.

Science can therefore be mistaken. Bad science is particularly prone to making mistakes when based upon false assumptions and preconception. However, the good thing about science is it is constantly progressing and dismissing false beliefs based on findings.

Furthermore, science is never based on just one single research project. Often these days, when reading the daily newspaper or listening to your favorite radio host giving everyone a lesson, you hear the phrase *research shows* – which is now considered as the single most sacred truth. These vague and false assumptions are then usually reinforced with the opinion of an "expert" who appears on TV promising spectacular results and fairytales and with that this fiction soon becomes a topic of everyone's conversation on Facebook. And if something appears on Facebook *and* on TV, any existing doubts immediately disappear. Because it gets considered as fact.

Unfortunately, it isn't so. We can speak of science whenever a theory has been proven multiple times through various independent types of research and in different labs, involving large amounts of test subjects and using measures that allow experiments to be repeatable and give identical or consistent results. Real science rarely makes its way to Facebook or appears on TV because all relevant scientific findings take time for reflection and peer review and most of all require understanding. This means not only being able to follow the letters of an article, but understand precisely the conclusions it reaches and be familiar with the procedures and methods used in scientific research.

It's also worth knowing that science is mostly presented by using percentages and probability. For example, a certain percentage of test subjects showed that this method works in this particular way. Even medication prescribed to you by a doctor may not be effective for you. Some individuals won't relieve their headache by taking aspirin, but the aspirin will instead upset their stomach.

However, this doesn't mean that aspirin isn't effective against headache. While it is effective for a large percentage of people, exceptions still exist.

It is therefore important you don't fall for it whenever you come across the overused term "research shows". It is more than likely that the person making the claims doesn't know what kind of research they are describing, where it was published and what the results actually showed. When it comes to weight loss methods, hearing the phrase "research shows" usually indicates you need to start protecting your wallet.

This is exactly what we are trying to protect you from with this book. We are going to use simple and comprehensive ways to introduce you to the existing trends based on the research involving the low intake of carbohydrates and high intake of fats; none of it is far-fetched but presents current scientific conclusions. These findings have been beneficial to countless people all over the world by either helping them change the composition of their body or assisting them in relieving the symptoms of a medical condition. But science is forever evolving. Most research indicates that additional research is necessary.

An initial piece of advice from us would be to listen to yourself and your body. My co-author's body, for instance, is constantly throwing tantrums, it rejects exercise, craves copious amounts of pizza and chocolate, even smoking, and prefers to be about as active as a dysfunctional fat blob. But we're not talking about that voice: we urge you to try and find an inner voice that craves well-being, a relaxing inner sense of the body, clear thoughts, pleasure, calmness and health. This voice exists in each and every one of us. You need to become familiar with this voice, despite it being overwhelmed by the internalized hysterical TV screaming, online click baiting and greedy sales pitches from people who see nothing more than an on opportunity to profit from your issues. Get to know yourself.

On Choice of Words and other Semantic Affairs

Fats
This book contains a lot of information about dietary fat. Fats can be tricky and confusing, since we need to know what kind of fat we are talking about. When describing carbohydrates or protein, there is no confusion as it is generally understood we're describing food and not parts of our body. Our bodies contain carbohydrates, but we use the terms glucose and glycogen. At the same time there are large portions of our body consisting of protein, but they are once again generally given specific names such as muscle or lean tissue.

This is not the case with fats. We distinguish a fatty steak and a fatty butt (the human butt, not the butt of the animal the steak came from). Therefore, we should always acknowledge the difference between *dietary* fat and *body* fat. The latter can then be divided further into blood fat, fat deposits in the hypodermis and other parts and the fat that present in organs, tissues and cells. In laboratories, blood fat is more commonly known as blood lipids and your doctor may call your "love handles" adipose tissue or subcutaneous fat.

Healthy and Natural
Don't get us wrong, but when it comes to healthy foods, or the advantages of natural foods, any kind of debate is pointless: speaking either of "healthy foods" or superiority

of "natural whatever" is a C short of crime and should be prosecuted by the common sense police.

There are no healthy foods, or as the former Slovenian nutritionist Dr. Drazigost Pokorn stated – there are only healthy meal plans and healthy dietary regimens. At the same time things aren't necessarily better just because they are natural. Arsenic is fully natural, but instead of being good, healthy or useful, it is toxic. Some pesticides can also be "natural" and at the same time more toxic than synthetic pesticides.

This sort of imposed duality often leads to the creation of false conceptions about certain foods and nutrients. And one of those misconceptions is that fats are unhealthy. The truth is out there, mocking us and thinking to itself: it's all relative, everything changes, fat simply remains fat. Fats come in a variety of forms, each with different chemical structures which determine their specific roles in the body.

As a side note: a large majority of dietary fats are natural. We will help you avoid synthetic fats that are found in processed foods.

"Porklings"

The book was originally written in a local language with local food in mind. We had quite some issues with a specific pork lard product, locally called *ocvirki*. There are many varieties of the dish and hence many different names: pork cracklings or cracklins, pork greaves, pork scratchings, scrunchions, grattons or pork rinds. These however do not describe the same things: some include pork skin, some don't. Some are combination of pork fat and skin. Then there are some that are made out of bacon (they include meaty parts) and some that consist just of the unmeltable residue left after animal fat has been rendered. Basically, it's just the lard, cut in blocks of about an inch, slowly fried in its own fat until crispy.

The translator and authors had discussions with native speakers from Canada, US and the UK – each of them having their own idea about how these should be called. We decided to go for pork cracklings – but you might as well prefer to munch on pork rinds. We love those as well!

Diets

We encountered a few dilemmas we'd like to point out regarding the terms for dietary regimens described in this book, in order to avoid any misunderstandings and bickering.

The co-author prefers to use the term dietary regimen instead of a diet. The reason behind this is that in informal conversations the term diet carries a negative or a temporary meaning. We usually "start a diet" and eventually, when we reach our goals, we stop and "finish a diet". The diet is temporary as it is hard work and requires a lot of sacrifice and distress.

None of that is implied regarding the dietary regimens we present. No high-fat intake diet (common ketogenic or less strict type of a LCHF diet) is set out as a short-term summer adventure that will raise your levels of oxytocin and other "happy hormones" and will then let you return to your abusive partner. On the contrary: the plan is for a dietary regimen rich in fats to become a sustainable, comfortable and beneficial change of dietary habits. For this reason it would indeed be better to use the term "dietary regimen", nevertheless, the decision to use the term "diet" was made.

It's also worth explaining the relation and the difference between the terms ketogenic diet and the LCHF diet. More often than not, the term LCHF is considered as a generally used term for dietary regimens that include a more or less dramatic **limited intake of carbohydrates and protein, while increasing the fat intake**. Scientific publications sometimes use the abbreviation LCKD (*Low Carb Ketogenic Diet* – a ketogenic diet with a very low intake of carbohydrates). When describing the LCHF diet in this book, we are talking about a diet that involves a very low consumption of carbohydrates and a very high consumption of fats. This means a diet with a daily intake of up to 50 to 100 grams of carbohydrates, or a quarter of a daily energy intake.

When using the term ketogenic diet, we generally think of the **standard ketogenic diet** with a strictly minimal carbohydrate intake. This diet consists of a daily consumption of 20–50 grams of carbohydrates, or approximately 5 to 10 percent of daily energy intake. In addition to the phrase ketogenic diet, we sometimes use the term fat rich diet. Scientific publications name this strict version of the diet VLCKD (*Very Low Carb Ketogenic Diet* – ketogenic diet with **very** low carbohydrate intake).

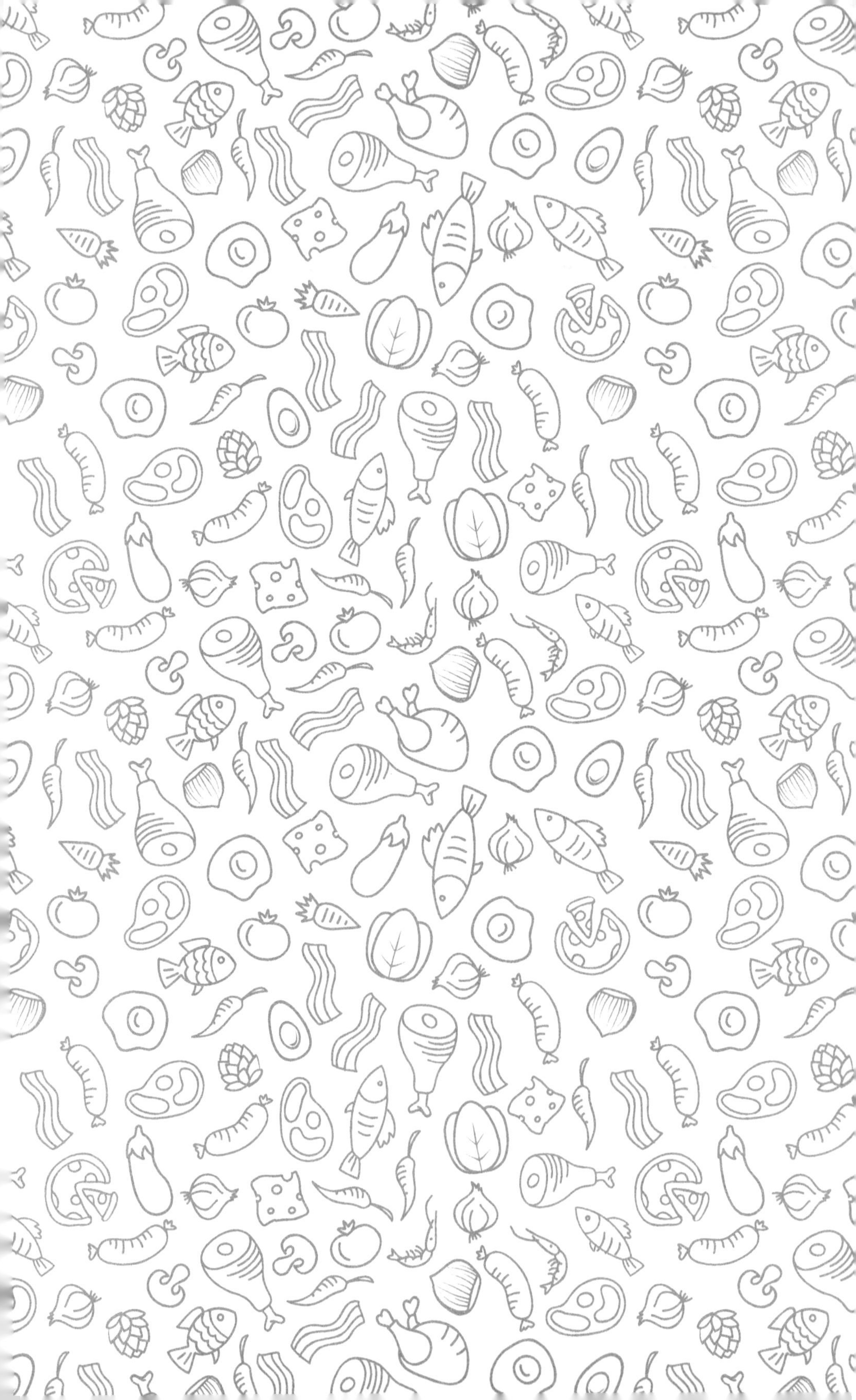

FAT IN THE 21ST CENTURY: PUBLIC ENEMY NUMBER 1

How Did We Manage to Get So Fat?

In 1980 the American government first published a dietary guidelines document, which had a distinct effect on dietary habits throughout the modern world. Among other recommendations they suggested a restricted intake of total fats, saturated fats and cholesterol, a sufficient intake of starchy foods and fiber, avoiding sugar and salt, and using alcohol in moderation .

While the intentions were likely positive, the recommendations unfortunately haven't brought the desired results, quite the contrary: they led to a complete disaster.

The World Health Organization (WHO) reports show the number of overweight and obese people in the world since 1980 has more than doubled. In 2014, there were 1.9 billion people in the world who were older than 18 and were classed as overweight, while 600 million of them were obese. This means that 39 percent of the people in this world (38 percent of men and 40 percent of women) were overweight, of which 13 percent were obese. In 2013, 42 million children under the age of 5 were considered overweight.

The majority of the world population lives in countries where more people die due to obesity than because of malnutrition.

Similar figures were presented in the European Union, with the only difference being a higher ratio of obesity among the male population. The percentage of the adult population in various countries, between the age of 25 and 64, considered either overweight or obese, ranges from 37 to 57 percent in women and 51 to 69 percent in men. Eurostat data produced interesting findings of obesity being inversely proportionate with education among the female population: meaning, the higher their education, the less likely it was for women to be obese. The same correlation could not be found among the male population.

Things look even worse in the US: while the overweight and obese in 1990 presented less than 15 percent of the entire population, today they represent a staggering 69 percent, with 36 percent of those considered obese.

We rarely reflect on this, but we take too many things for granted: stepping into a supermarket or ordering that mouthwatering pizza delivered to you by a dude on a moped, is not so "normal" or self-explanatory if you think about it. Having an easy way of obtaining food and having abundance of it, is – in the perspective of history – highly unusual and the time-span of this happening is relatively short. Unlike the past few decades, humans throughout history spent most of their time looking for food and making sure they got enough of it for themselves and their family. Food wasn't something they could take for granted, nor was it easily obtainable. Not only that, food shortage was almost always an issue.

Many theories found in dietary literature try to explain the reasons for the modern epidemic of obesity. This isn't just vanity: it's not simply about us dreaming of toned bodies like those seen on the covers of magazines, in movies and on TV. The presented statistics evidently show that most us are *actually* overweight. Unfortunately, being overweight is usually manifested as obesity of the central part of the body. It's called abdominal obesity and it isn't just an aesthetic issue, but a health issue that not only requires the attention of fitness coaches, but of all public health institutions around the world.

★ *To evaluate overweight and obesity, all public health institutions around the world use the Quetelet index, named after the 19th century Belgian mathematician and astronomer. Today it is known as the body mass index (BMI). BMI is a function of body weight expressed in kilograms and height expressed in meters (BMI is the body weight divided with the square of the height). Despite the fact that BMI isn't the best reference point, since it doesn't tell us anything about the composition of the body, it is still quite useful when studying nutrition among the population. In order to be able to perform any kind of decent evaluation of an individual's condition, it is necessary to take into account the waist circumference and other indicators (blood triglycerides levels, potential incidence of type 2 diabetes, etc.).*

★ *If you'd like to learn more about the unreliability of the BMI, we recommend the book Fat Politics, written by J. Eric Oliver.*

Why Are You Overweight?

You probably don't hear that often, but before making any kind of changes to your diet or way of living, we kindly recommend you think about the reasons for your obesity and overnutrition.

Do you eat more because of stress, do you lack the time to spend on yourself because of an important job role, or do you take care of all your family members (despite them being capable of taking care of themselves, but it just feels good to know you are indispensable)? Is it never the right time to deal with your obesity, because of an exam or a work project? Does it run in your family and is it genetic by nature? Are you big-boned? Are you having issues with your thyroid gland? Are you obese because of medication? Do you hardly eat anything, yet every little thing you do eat shows on your hips? Are your metabolism and digestion slow?

Give it a second thought!

Let us help by saying: it is never the right time to work on yourself. But nonetheless, any moment is more than appropriate to start taking care of yourself. Taking care of your excess fat deposits can be a matter of vanity, but being slimmer will expand your lifespan so there's many more years for you to be stressed out, keep yourself even busier and be able to take care of your family members, who are ignorant of your hard work for as long as they're comfortable.

Also, it will help you remain indispensable at work, where they will surely build a monument with your name on it, on the piece of grass outside your office, to thank you for your input. It's a win-win situation, right?

Does this sound like we're messing with you? We're not, we're trying to tell that the reasons for your obesity are nothing but excuses without any logic behind them. It is almost always the case that we try to attribute excess fat to other things, circumstances, as long we avoid admitting to ourselves that we're the only ones responsible. We all do this; therefore we strongly urge you to think about yourself: do that sincerely and without suppressing anything. Social obligations, commercial pressure and social conventions make us more susceptible to mistakes, but if these obligations, pressure and conventions were to suggest you punch yourself in the face, you would most probably respond: "Hm. No, thanks, maybe some other time."

If everyone in your family is obese, then the reason for that might be bad nutritional habits and a lack of physical activity. Although your aunt sometimes gets on your nerves and you hardly have anything in common with her, you most likely have similar dietary habits, because people adopt most of their dietary habits from their close family and therefore "obesity becomes inherited". Yes, we all just might have that evil gene for obesity, but it is only expressed in environments that support it. No gene will make you fat if there is a shortage of food in your environment. You could be big-boned, have a wide frame, it is possible, but still isn't related to that soft cushion you have grown between your ribs and pelvis. Those aren't bones. That's lard.

Some people are obese because of problems with their thyroid gland. That's serious shit and nothing to joke about. The problem is that 99 percent of those who *claim* to have "thyroid gland problems" don't really have any problems with it, but happily convince themselves that the reason for their excess fat deposits are in no way related to their awful dietary habits and sedentary life-style. Sometimes, both reasons go hand in hand.

The same goes for medication. Some medications affect the appetite and other processes in the body that lead to storing fat. But medication can't be blamed for your obesity if all you ever do is lay on the couch and stuff yourself with sweets and potato chips. There isn't a medication out there capable of going to the shop and bringing you the unhealthiest snacks.

You may be a person with a slow metabolism, but the speed and efficiency of your metabolism are not set in stone – what's more, it seems that slow metabolism, or low basal metabolic rate, is not necessarily a factor of a potential weight gain or obesity [2]. People vary: some pass math exams with last minute study marathons, others by constant retaking of exams.

One way or another, anyone who values themselves and their education is forced to tackle mathematical questions successfully to pass.

Metabolism works in a similar way: if you're a male in your 20s, your metabolism acceleration, compared to that of a 40-year-old chubby woman, is distinctly better. But does this mean that middle aged women should throw in the towel? Of course not. But you could use your circumstances as an excuse for your laziness and lack of motivation. That's fine. None of us make it out of this life alive anyway. You just happen to be an all-consuming eater and you would rather not worry about your health too much. Even this kind of attitude towards health has its advantages. Maybe you will make it to 90 years of age with your 260 lbs and maybe, even at that age, you will still be able to move around normally despite those 260 lbs. Although possible, it's highly unlikely.

History Of Food Consumption

We understand how you feel: every piece of pie that you guiltily swallow attaches itself to your hips, your stomach, or ends up as fat that decorates your triceps. From an evolutionary point of view, you are a winner. We've mentioned earlier that throughout human history, food supply was extremely scarce. Our ancestors experienced short periods with an abundance of food and longer periods when it was very hard to come by. Therefore, to survive, evolutionary adaptation made perfect sense, creating as large an amount of fat deposits as possible, from as little food as possible, which then serve as energy in periods when food isn't available. In harsh prehistoric circumstances, the ability to store energy from a low intake of food proved to be a survival advantage.

Even though every apple that passes by your mouth, affects your figure, as far as natural selection is concerned, you are still an advanced model. You are adjusted, improved. People with fast and immaculate metabolisms have fought through the evolutionary process by sheer luck, while the rest of us were given a better chance of survival through DNA.

Today, this excellent explanation is neither useful nor comforting, since food shortages never occur and we're instead fighting issues created by a surplus of food.

But despite having these fat storing abilities long before the modern era, overweight and obesity are more or less 150 to 200 year old problems, which in recent decades became not only a problem for individuals, but almost an epidemic.

How did this happen?

We all carry our own bit of responsibility for having a bad body composition, but the factors affecting the extent of the obesity related issues are evidently systemic and relatively easy to define in terms of human history. To simplify, the history of human food consumption can roughly be divided into four key time periods:

- prehistory;
- Neolithic and the periods following the agricultural revolutions;
- period following the industrial revolution;
- period from 1952 onward.

Prehistoric Period Before the Neolithic Revolution

For the greater part of human history, humans fed themselves the same way as their ancestors: they picked plants and fruit and hunted animals, they consumed what nature offered without being able to influence it in any way.

History shows that local tribes were usually dependent on around ten or fifteen types of free-growing plants and free-living animals. Hunter-gatherers were nomads, who traveled to obtain food and had no particular reason to settle anywhere permanently. They had less children, since nomad life without a cart wasn't very comfortable. Reproduction was usually regulated with longer periods of breastfeeding, abstinence and even infanticide. In the Stone Age, when humans learned how to make tools out of stone, they used pear shaped sharp rocks to slaughter animals and to dig out the tasty edible roots, while they also enjoyed fruit, berries, nuts and grass. They hunted and killed large animals and usually used all of it – from entrails to brain. The least appetizing for the Stone age man was white, lean meat, which he sometimes left for other beasts to enjoy.

We are not wrong when we assume that people in those times didn't consume many carbohydrates– they were consumed rarely, when they were available. There was also hardly any starch and no refined sugar in their diet with the exception of honey, which humans always loved. There is also a lot of speculation regarding the protein to fat ratio in that period of time. Historians haven't made any definite conclusions about this subject yet.

To this day historiography and evolutionary anthropology still try to explain the reasons behind the sudden growth of the brain, which occurred a little under two million years ago. The volume of the brain of the homo habilis was around 600 ml, a million years later the volume of the brain of the homo erectus was approximately 900 ml, the homo sapiens' brain measured 1200 ml, while the homo sapiens sapiens' brain measured approximately 1400 ml. Most theories connected with brain growth correlate this with dietary changes, while some scientist even claim the growth itself was a result of the consumption of fat-rich meat. A group of Israeli scientists claims that the first major growth of the human brain (even the homo habilis had a larger brain than the simians before them) came at a price. Because brain function required a lot of energy, the digestive system got shorter and the organism became dependent on energy rich foods. As described in a paper, published in the journal PLOS ONE in 2011, "it would therefore appear that it was the human carnivorousness rather than herbivorous nature that most probably energized the process of encephalization through-out most of human history" [3].

The Neolithic Agricultural Revolutions
The last ice age ended around 16,000 BC. Global warming resulted in increased precipitation, creating ideal conditions for a type of wild weed to evolve, a plant already known to man, but only occasionally consumed; wheat. It wasn't an overnight process, but with time humans

abandoned nomad life because of wheat and other crops. This agricultural revolution occurred almost "simultaneously" in numerous places on Earth between the years 9,000 and 5,000 BC. Considering the entire 2.5 million years of human history this practically happened yesterday. Well, about 15 minutes ago.

> ★ *Most common beliefs claim that the agricultural revolution began on the Fertile Crescent in the Middle East, but we know today that the agriculture sprang up entirely independently in many parts of the world.*

By gradually settling and getting accustomed to livestock farming and agriculture, humans experienced a lot of struggle and their lives were far from comfortable. The abundance of food we have today remained just a dream for most the human race for thousands of years. Obesity didn't exist and if it did, it was highly valued: it was admired by artists depicting people's bodies and faces and it was also valued from the medical perspective of that time.

The Industrial Revolution
Overweight and obesity fully began appearing after the technological and social progress triggered by the industrial revolution. The industrial revolution brought changes into every little part of individual human life and into society itself. We can compare the processes of the first two industrial revolutions in the mid 18th and 19th century, which changed human life as drastically as the agricultural revolution in the Mid-Neolithic, 10,000 years ago.

Compared to the agricultural revolution, which didn't improve the quality of human life and people's well-being by much (according to numerous authors it even made things worse), the industrial revolution was different:

while the changes weren't instantaneous, there was still, for the first time ever in history, an improvement in the standard of living for the general population.

For the first time ever, obesity became a problem – a merely aesthetic one at the time. Gradually, the constant shortage of food from which humans suffered up until the 19th century became a thing of the past and food was permanently available for a large portion of society, not just the privileged at the top of the political leadership hierarchy.

The accessibility of food wasn't just a case of supply exceeding demand. Today's supermarket "hunter-gatherers" existence is based on a range of technological advances in preservation, freezing and cooling technology and transport logistics.

It's been more than 200 years since the invention of the tin can, which like many other important inventions was created for the military, during the Napoleonic Wars. During their advances far east, Napoleon's army was looking for a cheap and efficient way of storing large quantities of food. The first of the food preservation methods involved the use of airtight jars, but glass soon proved to be a very impractical material for the army, therefore in 1810 Peter Durand introduced a preservation method using galvanized steel containers. Over the next few decades the tin can was perfected and by the mid-19th century it became a very important household novelty and was already commercially available through many companies.

The other fundamental innovation on which today's food supply is based today is deep-freezing. Humans tried freezing their food long before, but their methods weren't nor reliable neither rapid enough: the frozen food would lose its flavor and texture. Modern freezing methods were adopted from the Inuit, who freeze their fish quickly and to very low temperatures. Once this distinction between freezing the food slowly and freezing it rapidly was understood, the invention of a device that would replicate the Inuit freezing techniques, was just around the corner.

The 20th century brought some truly dramatic changes: self-service supermarkets growing into large commercial chains; in 1929 we saw the appearance of the first ever efficient freezer; a year later the electric oven was invented. The shopping cart is an invention originating from the late 30s of the previous century. In the same period, refrigerators and freezers became common household items and deep frozen food was first considered an important part of the store supply.

The economic crisis of the 30s, at least in the US, brought some very important measures: because of a demand for large quantities of energy rich food, the American Congress brought in measures to subsidize the cultivation of industrial and farm crops, mostly corn and soybeans. These measures remain effective to this day, therefore it's no surprise that the huge agricultural conglomerates, which in recent decades took over almost the entire crop farming, are using all means necessary to make sure their already subsidized produce gets used in abnormal circumstances. Using high fructose corn syrup in obnoxious amounts in all types of food products (drinks, sweets, even for glazing fruit, etc.), huge marketing campaigns and efforts for promoting soy as a supposed superfood – all of this originates from the support policies, which might have made sense during the cruel economic crisis, but today represent one of the factors for human dietary struggles.

Urbanization, which began shortly after the industrial revolution and all its drastic changes in agricultural mechanization, was spreading unprecedentedly after the Second World War. For the first time in human history, people didn't produce their food with their own hands anymore, but increasingly began shopping for it.

Towards the end of the 40s there was another significant change: the invention of the first efficient refrigerated truck, which enabled the transportation of food over long distances. Up to that moment it was common for people to eat locally produced and processed food, but with the introduction of refrigerated trucks, it was suddenly possible to transport food far from the place where it was produced.

The post war decades brought many more advances in the cultivation technology, processing, transport and perception of food itself, which forever marked people's dietary habits: from the fast food industry to the microwave oven, and the development of cultural trends such as eating out and so on.

As the side effect of all these lifestyle and dietary changes, an increase in excess body weight and even obesity became apparent: people simply needed a much smaller energy input in order to get their hands on enough food for themselves and their families and, unlike before the industrial revolution, everything was made accessible and affordable.

Obesity Epidemic and Measures to Control it

Obesity, these days often labeled using the terms "overweight and obesity", was first considered a medical problem towards the end of the 18th century, yet everyone believed carrying 20 to 40 extra pounds was a sign of vitality and good health far into the 19th century.

All of that changed in the 1930s. Medicine shifted its opinion and excess "meat" slowly became a medical issue.

It's funny, and at the same time interesting, that the origin of this transition comes from a rather unusual place: the insurance industry. Because there were no useful mechanisms for determining the risks of disease and mortality at the beginning of the 20th century, Louis I. Dublin, a statistician and a vice president of the insurance company *Metropolitan Life Insurance Company*, made the decision to rely– as always – on statistics. He was able to establish that insurance holders who were overweight tended to die younger due to obesity or other related specific diseases. He compared the ratio between body height, body weight and mortality and discovered that the closer the body weight of a person is to the bodyweight of an average 25 year old person, the longer that person would most likely live. In short, slimmer people statistically live longer. He created probability tables called *Met Life* that were based on his own statistical analysis and, along with the acknowledgment of obesity as a problem, became publicly used: they were used by doctors, epidemiologists and policy makers. When it came to determining the level of overweight and obesity, those tables were considered almost as sacred all the way to the 1950s.

After the First World War and in the 1930s there was an increase of people suffering from cardiac arrest. This totally new development started to upset the public. Scary situations are still welcomed by potential saviors, people driven by an overwhelming ambition to find the magic cure or indisputable explanation, who would be followed by crowds of believers. Quite often – even today – these kinds of people have no restraints when it comes to using science, expert terminology and their own authority to fulfill their ambition.

But as history showed us numerous times before, abusing scientific authority and desperately gathering evidence to support a certain theory, while simultaneously ignoring all opposing claims, can do a lot of damage that is hard to repair. In the current internet era, these sensationalisms are igniting and spreading online like wildfire through dry summer bushes, and more substantially than they did in the 1950s. But even then, pseudo-science was similarly based on nonsense and despite having good intentions, it created a complete and big fat mess.

What actually happened?

Disguised as objective science, superstition and false beliefs made their way into medical research. You've probably heard the saying "you are what you eat". This kind of belief is outdated and ridiculous: ancient warriors often believed that by consuming the flesh of certain types of animals they would acquire their characteristics. In their desire to be faster they consumed the claws of fast and agile hunters, bear paws for strength and tiger penis and blood for boosting libido. You most probably think these sort of beliefs are deceiving and highly unbeliev-able, yet even today literal understanding of the maxim "you are what you eat" is still one of the most common misconceptions. By consuming radioactive uranium, you unfortunately won't become a nuclear plant, but just a pile of radioactive biological waste. For the same reasons, someone who eats a lot of bread and cake won't turn into a walking loaf.

One of the elemental beliefs from the "you are what you eat" category is that dietary fats turn into body fat, or to cut it short: fats make you fat.

This was "proven" true on numerous times by Dr. Ancel Benjamin Keys from the University of Minnesota. Dr. Keys identified the culprit that was behind the increasing rates of obesity, performed a few studies using questionable data which may have proven his idea and the rest became the history of the obesity epidemic, which he was to tackle with his published "scientific" contribution.

> ★ *Dr. Keys' beliefs were borderline magic and far from original: an ancient Greek healer name Galen believed people can get rid of excess weight by consuming the flesh of lean, predominantly wild animals. Numerous medieval healers believed that by consuming pork, people would become gluttonous like pigs. A common misconception regarding the behavior of fats inside and outside of the body, when we hear people today speak about a certain food's "fat melting" abilities, is a similar kind of false belief. The fat in our body does not melt. Body fat would burn if the individual was put in a furnace, but that wouldn't be very healthy and would dramatically shorten their lifetime to a few difficult and excruciating minutes.*

Dr. Keys is considered the author of the so called diet-heart hypothesis: fat consumption leads to high cholesterol, which then leads to atherosclerosis which then causes cardiovascular disease. He first introduced this hypothesis in 1952. Creating the hypothesis is not objectionable – many scientific theories and hypotheses are examined and discarded. The main issue with Dr. Keys' heritage is the fact that the data confirming his hypothesis was acquired selectively and some parts of his own research were ignored, so they wouldn't undermine his narrative. Instead of doing the reasonable thing by discarding his conjecture, like a meticulous gardener he cut away all the ugly pieces that didn't look pretty in his rose garden. And what he cut off wasn't just weed.

Many of the researchers who found errors in his research and conclusions tried to make him acknowledge the inaccurate conclusions, yet were unsuccessful, since Dr. Keys arrogantly and aggressively defended his savior theory. One of his main opponents was the British doctor John Yudkin, who in 1957 in the magazine The Lancet, first published a hypothesis suggesting sugar might be to blame for the modern world's obesity problems, a food used for only a few hundred years and only more commonly used within the last century. Statistics were pointing the blame for cardiovascular disease at sugar, as was good old common sense: why would fats all of a sudden be harmful to us, if we managed to consume them without any issues during the majority of our evolution?

Unfortunately, in the following decades Dr. Yudkin didn't get to defend his case against an onslaught of aggressive overambitious researchers and public policy makers in the field of human nutrition and industry. Dr. Keys fought against him impetuously using generalized judgments. The sugar industry, once they could smell blood, also jumped in on the action. Dr. Yudkin later quietly passed away and it wasn't until recent years that his work has again been revived.

Dr. Keys was known mostly by two studies: "six countries study" (published title *Atherosclerosis: A problem in newer public health* from 1953 [4]) and "seven countries study" (starting in 1958 and lasting over 50 years [5]). The first of his two studies, claiming fat consumption leads to cardiovascular disease, was validated using data from six countries, showing the presence of a distinctive statistical correlation between high fat intake and cardiovascular disease. But although he had data from 22 countries, he only took 6 into account. Which were only those confirming his "fat is bad" narrative.

For the "seven countries study" he carefully decided which countries to pick after clearly giving it a lot of thought. No harm in that, you might say. In science, picking a representative and random study sample is very important. If we want to prove that all tables are made out of laminated paperboard, we select a sample consisting of 5 stores from the same Swedish manufacturer – *et voilà*: all tables are made out of laminated paperboard. That's exactly what Keys did. And that isn't good science.

Amongst others discrepancies in the "seven countries study" he, for example, performed studies of the population of Crete, where people are known for their longevity, which is allegedly down to their low fat intake, but the studies were performed at a time period when they were still recovering from war and fasting, during which, of course, they didn't consume meat and cheese. That still isn't good science.

All of this shouldn't have been more than a sidebar of dietary history, but Dr. Keys was incredibly ambitious and convincing. Because of his connections in important organizations, he was able to disseminate his "findings" for decades before any doubts appeared, and despite cardiovascular disease and obesity still being present today, many still presume they are best avoided by not consuming fat rich foods.

Dietary guidelines in the majority of countries, including member states of the EU, are based upon Keys' poor conclusions regarding causes and effects. Even though Dr. Keys, his associates, students and successors might have had good intentions, they dragged us into an epidemic of poor health, overnutrition, obesity, cardiovascular disease, diabetes and metabolic syndrome. Obviously, the food industry and its interests made matters worse by offering goods that were easy to sell, and if this meant selling carbohydrates, then so be it. If a large demand for non-fat (but sugarcoated) yogurt appears, they meet that demand.

The only goal of traders and suppliers are sales. It's even easier for them to achieve that goal if something happens to be an official public health dogma. Traders would definitely be willing to supply you with uranium if you desired to become a nuclear plant, but since that's illegal it's out of the question. We have already mentioned a large number of other factors that made matters worse in the current obesity epidemic: the continuation of urbanization, motorization, commercializing of dietary habits, a distinctive transition from home cooking to eating out, sedentary lifestyle and many others.

It was only in the last 15 years that slow and gradual changes in the attitude and behavior regarding the role of fats in the human diet started appearing and claims were made, suggesting that stuffing yourself with carbohydrates to the extent proposed by the public health organizations may be an awful idea.

That is also the reason why you will hear of the low carb-high fat diet only from the "heretics who do not believe in the holy war against the damned fat". The official dogma still exists and claims we should get our energy predominantly from the carbohydrates. The changing of official dogmas is a slow process: we shouldn't expect the governmental Departments of Health to suddenly flip the record over. As a matter of fact, this is how it should be: as mentioned before, science is never quick. Science requires the accumulation of knowledge, double checking of theories, proving and studying – all of which demands time and funds.

We would absolutely love to be able to say: we've got it! We've got the magic bullet against obesity, cardiovascular disease, diabetes, metabolic syndrome, autoimmune disease and, if possible, against stupidity and narrow-mindedness. Plus a proof it works with a few little short studies involving 500 people. Sadly, that isn't the case. The dietary approach in which we drastically lower the intake of carbohydrates and increase the intake of fats shows good results, but it is, to use a bit of sports slang, just at "the intermediate time point". The finish line is still a long way ahead.

THEORY

How does Our Body Get Energy from Food?

The human body needs energy to function (among other things). But for now let's focus on energy, as the choice of type of primary energy source is what distinguishes low-carb diets from all other diets.

The human organism is a complex structure which, through the process of evolution, developed many defense mechanisms. One of these mechanisms is the ability to run on different types of fuel.

Unlike cars, where it's not a good idea to put gasoline in a diesel engine, the human body is far more adaptable. If it runs out of gasoline, it starts using diesel, it can also run on energy from the battery, use gas and even electricity from the grid. To sum it up, the human body is a fantastic hybrid machine, capable of functioning on three main groups of nutrients, regardless of the food intake ratio.

But just because it can function like that doesn't necessarily mean that all types of food combinations are optimal. Today this has become the topic of various doctrines and emerging theories. At the current time the leading doctrine still states that the most optimal fuel for the human body is glucose. Since carbohydrates are built from units of glucose, the body simply breaks it down into readily available energy. The influx of glucose replenishes glycogen stored in the liver and muscles. Whenever those are full, the liver magically transforms glucose into fatty acids, which then travel through the bloodstream and get stored for times of shortage – in form of body fat. Unlike protein and fats, none of the carbohydrates are essential: they are not a mandatory part of our diet, since if it's an emergency, our body knows how to create glucose out of certain parts of fat and amino acids.

Proteins provide substances for the human body, which it essentially needs for creating its own protein (for example, but not only, muscles) and other substances. In some cases, the body is able to use protein as an energy source: consumed protein (in desperate times of starvation even body protein) transforms into glucose. We call this process gluconeogenesis and it can also occur as a result of an excess protein intake. When there is no need for amino acids, which protein usually breaks down to, the body transforms these amino acids into glucose. And in extreme cases, even this excess of glucose will end up in body's energy storage, which we fondly refer to by different cute names such as love handles, muffin top, potbelly or a spare tire.

The third source our body is capable of using as energy, are dietary and body fats. In our body, fats just like protein have several different functions. The most obvious of those is being the energy source, but they also play many other important physiological and structural roles: they are components of cellular membranes, nerves, organs, building blocks of hormones, they are a part of the immune system and numerous other molecules with significant body functions, they are also vital for metabolism and providing vitamins A, D, E and K. Any excessive decrease in the amount of consumed fats can trigger issues in all of the described processes.

Different cell types can use different energy sources. Some cannot use fatty acids and ketones, therefore they urgently require glucose. This function is predominantly determined by the amount of mitochondria in the cells:

• cells with a lot of mitochondria (skeletal muscles, heart muscle) will in times of shortage of glucose, use mostly fats – in form of fatty acids;

• cells that have a lot of mitochondria but are unable to use fatty acids (central nervous system, brain) will in times of shortage of glucose use mostly ketones to function;

• cells with very few or even without any mitochondria (red cells, medulla, eye lens and retina, testicles) urgently need glucose.

Macronutrient	breaks down to:	used for:	in certain circumstances it is transformed into:
Carbohydrates	glucose	energy	fatty acids
Protein	amino acids	body structure and other processes	glucose, fatty acids
Fats	fatty acids, glycerol	energy, body structure and other processes	glucose

In case we don't consume enough carbohydrates through food, our body's adapted itself to produce glucose from glycerol (a component of fats), lactate and some amino acids.

Furthermore, glucose enters the brain independently of insulin. Approximately 60 percent of all of body's glucose is in the cerebrospinal fluid surrounding brain. Insulin's journey to the brain is not an easy one: the higher its blood concentration, the less of it makes it to the brain, especially when cells transporting it from blood to brain, due to constant insulin excess become immune to it. This can result in brain having glucose at its disposal, yet being unable to use it. Many studies in recent years acknowledge the importance of metabolic balance on the health of brain. The theory about Alzheimer's disease being in fact a disorder based on disruptions of insulin, glucose and the insulin-like growth factor (IGF-1) metabolism is gaining traction in the scientific community. Many even call it a type 3 diabetes.

Dietary Fats

If you intend to use the dietary fats as the energy substitute for carbohydrates, it most probably makes sense that you get familiar with them.

Newborn babies, breastfed by well-nourished mothers, get 50 to 60 percent of their energy from fats, including cholesterol. What is good for newborn babies is not necessarily good for adults, nevertheless, it remains a fact that sheds a different light on the present beliefs regarding fat consumption.

Dietary fats are organic substances, insoluble in water and rich in energy. As we mentioned earlier, they also play many other key roles in the human body and in this chapter we'll be focusing on describing what those are and what they do.

Most fats consumed by humans are animal fat and vegetable oils and come in form of *triglycerides*, consisting of molecules of three fatty acids and glycerol. During metabolism, these molecules usually break down to components, fatty acids and glycerol, which are more useful for the organism. Another important lipid we consume is *cholesterol*. Both types of lipids – triglycerides and cholesterol – are furthermore measured as blood lipids, while it's not necessary that the correlation between the amount of consumed dietary fats and the blood lipids profile exists.

That last sentence is very important. It represents everything we've believed in and internalized for decades and points to it being a mistake. In order to explain why many scientists think that fat rich diets are beneficial to blood lipid levels, it is worth remembering and refreshing our knowledge regarding what we consume when eating fats and how it affects our blood.

Triglycerides
Fats in food are stored in molecules called triglycerides (also named triacylglycerols or triacylglycerides, often shortened to TAG, or TG).

Triglycerides are the main components of fats (animal and human fat and vegetable oils). The name of the substance tells us there are three fatty acids joined together by glycerol. We distinguish triglycerides based on which fatty acids are attached to glycerol: they can be three of the same kind, or three different ones. These long chain molecules are an important energy source since they can be broken down into particular fatty acids and glycerol, which can then be used to produce glucose. Increased levels of triglycerides in blood are crucial factors for development of various types of disease – mainly atherosclerosis, cardiac arrest and type 2 diabetes. Most of triglycerides are transported through bloodstream by lipoprotein VLDL (more on this later, in the chapter on *Cholesterol*).

Fatty acids, the basic building block of fats, are chains of carbon and hydrogen, varying in length (we call these chains aliphatic chains) that are on one side attached to the carboxyl group (-COOH). The main differences between fatty acids are the characteristics of their chains, namely these two factors: saturation or unsaturation and length.

Degree of Saturation

To everyone less fond of chemistry, we suggest you try and think of a fatty acid as adults attached to ropes (carbon atom, C), where each adult holds one child in each hand (hydrogen atom, H) and the last adult in the chain has three children, while the first adult is pushing one child in a baby carriage (two oxygen atoms, O).

Saturated fatty acids are acids with all 4 of their bonds of individual carbon atoms in the aliphatic chain occupied: at the front and back carbon binds with the neighboring carbon atom and with one hydrogen atom per each side. The word saturation means that all bonding positions of an acid are fully occupied with hydrogen atoms and that there are single bonds between all atoms.

When bonding positions of fatty acids aren't fully occupied with hydrogen atoms and there are spare positions, we speak of unsaturated fatty acids. A chain of unsaturated fatty acids has got at least one carbon atom attached to one single hydrogen atom. The unoccupied slot is then used to connect with the neighboring carbon atom and form the "double" bond. If both sides of the double bond have hydrogen linked to carbon on the same side, we call this the cis configuration and if the hydrogen atoms are on opposite sides of each other, we call that the trans configuration, or trans-fatty acids.

Unsaturated fatty acids are classified into monounsaturated and polyunsaturated fatty acids. Monounsaturated fatty acids have only one carbon atom with one hydrogen atom and one double bond with the neighboring carbon atom, while polyunsaturated fatty acids have many carbon atoms like that. The number of missing hydrogen atoms corresponds with the number of double bonds. Although double bonds do not bend, the position of hydrogen atoms with the cis-configuration type of fatty acids does not make them straight, but mostly curved instead.

Let's try and imagine this in a more simple way again, just think of the saturated fat being a chain of adults with a child in each hand, whereas with the unsaturated fat, at least one of the adults in the chain holds just a single child, while using his unoccupied hand to connect with the adult in front of them.

Due to their typical chemical structure, saturated fatty acids are more resilient to oxidation and rancidity. They come in either solid or semi-solid form. The largest amount of saturated fatty acids is obtained from food of animal origin and from plant based oils that grow in hot climates – like coconut oil, for example.

Saturated fatty acids carry the worse reputation out of all fatty acids – and that is most likely unjustified. We most certainly know of their positive qualities: they're a part of cellular membrane, they maintain healthy bones, protect liver from certain toxins, they boost the immune system, help with the metabolism of essential fatty acids and are antimicrobial.

Monounsaturated fatty acids have a relatively stable chemical structure and can therefore be used in cooking as long as we don't burn them. It is certainly advisable to only heat fat as much as it is necessary. If possible, add most of them towards the end onto a hot dish, since by doing so, you preserve all of micronutrients.

Because of their unsaturated nature, the fatty acid molecules are somewhat curved: this is what keeps them in a liquid form at room temperature and turns them solid in colder temperatures. We obtain most of monounsaturated fats through foods such as: hazelnut, olive, avocado and almond oil, macadamia nuts, goose and duck fat, fish oil, hazelnuts.

Polyunsaturated fatty acids are unstable and therefore need to be stored accordingly in cool and dark places and they also aren't very suitable for any kind of cooking. For humans the most important polyunsaturated fatty acids are groups of fatty acids omega-6 and omega-3. Both of these groups contain one of the essential fatty acids, which we have to obtain through food, since our body can't produce it by itself: alpha-linolenic acid (omega-3) and linolenic acid (omega-6). Both play numerous vital roles in our body (cell membranes, hormone production, metabolism, memory and learning etc.), therefore it is crucial to include them in our diet. Same also goes for other fatty acids omega-3 and omega-6. Foods, the richest in polyunsaturated fats are: flaxseed, walnut, poppy seed, soy and corn oil, walnuts, sesame, fish oil.

It is strongly advisable to use fish (or fish oil) as the source of omega-3, since it contains fatty acids omega-3 DHA and EPA. Our body can produce both of these from alpha-linolenic acid (ALA), which can be obtained from flaxseed oil, but in that case they are synthesized in very small quantities, especially the DHA. It's interesting that the fatty acids omega-6 negatively affect the production of DHA from ALA, while saturated fatty acids promote it. On top of that, flaxseed oil is one of the most unstable oils and quickly becomes rancid and as such, can become toxic.

The numbers in the name of omega-3 or omega-6, tell us which consecutive carbon atom has a double bond on an unsaturated fatty acid, while the term omega marks the direction in which we count the atoms. We often mark this with the letter n-, for example n-3, or n-6. Omega-3 therefore means that the fatty acid has its first double bond on the third carbon atom, counting from the omega side of the fatty acid. All of the fatty acids have omega and delta sides. At the omega side of every fatty acid there is a methyl group -CH3, while the delta side has the carboxyl group -COOH.

You should be careful with polyunsaturated fats: obtaining enough omega-6 fatty acids is easy with today's foods, but there are not many omega-3 fatty acids, so regardless of your dietary regimen, it's worth ensuring a high enough intake of fish, or fish oil.

The ideal proportion between the omega-6 and omega-3 ranges between 1:1 or 2:1. This proportion (1:1) for instance, is that of free-range eggs, although free-range eggs with the proportion of 2.5:1 are considered as good. Eggs from cage farming have this proportion at approximately 13:1. The stereotypical Western supermarket diet the proportion of consumed omega-6 fatty acids and omega-3 acids, is shockingly bad: between 16:1 and 17:1.

The described differences in the structure of fatty acids determine their nature. However, food never contains just a single type of fatty acids: by saying that coconut oil is a source of saturated fatty acids, we simply imply this type is predominant. Each fatty food is composed of various parts of saturated and unsaturated fatty acids.

The Chain Length

Based on the length of the chains that form a particular fatty acid, they are further classified into short-chain, medium-chain, long-chain and very long-chain fatty acids. The number of carbon atoms in the chain determines the category of a fatty acid.

Short-chain fatty acids have less than 6 carbon atoms and are saturated, they are quickly absorbed in the gut and are consequently a good direct source of energy. Their antimicrobial nature is an important value. Short-chain fatty acids are capable of percolating the blood-brain barrier.

Medium-chain fatty acids have between 6 and 12 carbon atoms and are saturated and processed in a similar way to short-chain fatty acids. They're also important for the immune system and gut flora. We will cover medium-chain fatty acids in more detail later in the MCT *Oil* chapter.

Long-chain fatty acids have between 14 and 20 carbon atoms. They can be saturated, monounsaturated and poly-unsaturated, the two essential fatty acids are also among long-chain fatty acids. Long-chain fatty acids cannot be directly used as fuel, since they don't get absorbed directly in the gut, but instead go through a longer and more complex metabolic process. Very long-chain fatty acids consist of more than 22 carbon atoms.

All substances can be recorded and named in various ways and fatty acids are no exception. Some have general, trivial names (for example the butyric acid), all have systematic names (butyric acid is butanoic acid) and can be presented using either a molecular or a structural formula, or with a diagram.

In some situations, they will even be presented by a letter C (a chemical symbol for carbon) along with two numbers separated with a colon, for instance, C4:0. This type of record tells us that this is a fatty acid with 4 carbon atoms and with no existing double bonds, meaning this is a short-chain and saturated fatty acid. The record can appear also as 18:3 n-3, which means there are 18 carbon atoms, 3 double bonds and that the first of the two double bonds appears on the third carbon atom and we commonly describe this with the term "omega-3". Sometimes there are letters -t or -c next to these numbers: which describe either the trans or the cis configuration.

The Most Important Fatty Acids

The most common and the most important fatty acids for humans are presented in the table below.

trivial (chemical) name	the no. of C atoms; no. double bonds	saturation, -chain	sources
butyric (butanoic)	4; 0	saturated, short-	butter or milk fat
caproic (hexanoic)	6; 0	saturated, medium-	butter or milk fat, goat cheese
caprylic (octanoic)	8; 0	saturated, medium-	coconut oil
capric (decanoic)	10; 0	saturated, medium-	coconut oil
lauric (dodecanoic)	12; 0	saturated, medium-	coconut oil, African oil palm's kernels
myristic (tetradecanoic)	14; 0	saturated, long-	African oil palm's kernels, nutmeg, coconut oil
palmitic (hexadecanoic)	16; 0	saturated, long-	palm oil, pork, cocoa butter
stearic (octadecanoic)	18; 0	saturated, long-	shea butter, cocoa butter, fat derived from animals
arachidic (eicosanoic)	20; 0	saturated, long-	macadamia nuts, peanuts, hazelnuts

trivial (chemical) name	the no. of C atoms; no. double bonds	saturation, -chain	sources
behenic (docosanoic)	22; 0	saturated, very long-	peanuts, sunflower oil, soy oil, oilseed rape oil
lignoceric (tetracosanoic)	24; 0	saturated, very long-	peanuts, macadamia nuts, sunflower seeds, cashew nuts, small amount in most fat
myristoleic (9-tetradeceonic)	14; 1	monounsaturated, long-	certain types of Northern sea fish, some in beef, horse meat, poultry, butter and cream
palmitoleic (9-hexadecenoic)	16; 1	monounsaturated, long-	fish, macadamia nuts, most animal derived fat
oleic (9-octadecenoic)	18; 1	monounsaturated, long-	sunflower, olive, hazelnuts, almonds
ricinoleic (12-hydroxy-9-octadecenoic)	18; 1	monounsaturated, long-	castor oil, oilseed rape oil
vaccenic (11-octadecenoic)	18; 1	monounsaturated, long-	milk fat, fats from ruminant animals
gadoleic (9-eicosenoic)	20; 1	monounsaturated, long-	fish
erucic (13-docosenoic)	22; 1	monounsaturated, very long-	mustard oil, fish, rapeseed oil
linoleic (9,12-octadecadienoic) (LA)*	18; 2	polyunsaturated ω-6, long-	safflower, rapeseed, sunflower, walnut, poppy seed oil, oil from grape pips

trivial (chemical) name	the no. of C atoms; no. double bonds	saturation, -chain	sources
linolenic or alpha-linolenic (9,12,15-octadec-atrienoic) (ALA)*	18; 3	polyunsaturated ω-3, long-	rapeseed oil, flaxseed oil
gamma-linolenic (6,9,12-octadec-atrienoic) (GLA)	18; 3	polyunsaturated ω-6, long-	hemp, evening primrose, borage oil, oil from the seeds of blackcurrant
arachidonic (5,8,11,14-eicosa-tetraenoic) (AA)	20; 4	polyunsaturated ω-6, long-	fish, poultry, eggs, beef, sheep meat, pork
EPA (5,8,11,14,17-eicos-apentaenoic)	20; 5	polyunsaturated ω-3, long-	fish
DHA (4,7,10,13,16,19-doco-sahexaenoic)	22; 6	polyunsaturated ω-3, very long-	fish

Fatty Acid Profiles in Major Fatty Foods

As we already mentioned, fatty foods rarely consist of just one type of fatty acids. Quite the contrary: each food contains a wide range of various fatty acids – saturated and unsaturated, short-chain and long-chain. When we state that coconut oil is full of saturated fats, this means those are predominant in coconut oil and that there is less of other kind.

There is a list of fatty foods and their fatty acid profiles in the table below. Each column refers to the amount of individual fatty acids and the last column refers to the proportion between the omega-6 and omega-3. Any large content of omega-3 (second to last column) and a favorable proportion of omega-6 and omega-3 (the last column) is particularly emphasized. Ideal foods are marked with both the high content of omega-3 fatty acid and a favorable ratio of omega-6 and omega-3 (for example fish, fish oil, free-range eggs).

Type	SFA	MUFA	PUFA	CH	O6	O3	O6:O3
butter	51.4	21	3	215	2,728	315	8.66
Edam cheese	17.6	8.1	0.7	89	418	247	1.69
Emmental cheese	17.8	7.3	1	92	620	352	1.76
feta cheese	14.6	4.6	0.6	89	326	265	1.23
Gouda cheese	34.9	15.3	1.3	226	521	780	0.67
cream cheese	19.3	8.6	1.4	110	1,032	173	5.97
mozzarella fat (full fat)	13.2	6.6	0.8	79	393	372	1.06
Parmesan cheese	16.4	7.5	0.6	68	272	297	0.92
sour cream	11.5	5.1	0.8	52	625	83	7.53
fresh cream	23	10.7	1.4	137	836	538	1.55
peanut oil	16.9	46.2	32		32,005		
avocado oil	11.6	70.6	13.5		12,531	957	13.09
cocoa butter	60	32.9	3		2,800	100	28.00
coconut oil	85.2	6.6	1.7		1,800		
hemp oil	7	9	84		54,234	17,768	3.05
corn oil	12.7	24.7	54.7		53,510	1,161	46.09
flaxseed oil	9.4	20.2	66		12,701	53,304	0.24
hazelnut oil	7.4	78	10.2		10,101		
poppy seed oil	13.5	19.7	62.4		62,391		
almond oil	8.2	69.9	17.4		17,401		
olive oil	13.8	73	10.5		9,763	761	12.83
walnut oil	9.1	22.8	63.3		52,894	10,401	5.09
palm oil	49.3	37	9.3		9,100	200	45.50
sesame seed oil	14.2	39.7	41.7		41,304	300	137.68
soybean oil	15.6	22.8	57.7		50,422	6,789	7.43
sunflower oil	9.7	83.6	3.8		3,606	192	18.78
MCT oil	91.3	2.2	1		1,000		
rapeseed oil, rape-oil	7.4	63.3	28.1		18,645	9,138	2.04
hake	0.1	0.1	0.2	43	5	195	0.03
trout	0.7	1.1	1.2	59	239	812	0.29
crustaceans	0.3	0.3	0.7	152	28	540	0.05
fish oil (from cod liver)	23	47	23	570	935	19,736	0.05

Type	SFA	MUFA	PUFA	CH	O6	O3	O6:O3
sardines in oil	1.5	3.9	5.1	142	3,544	1,480	2.39
mackerel	3.3	5.5	3.3	70	219	2,670	0.08
tuna	0.2	0.2	0.3	45	8	243	0.03
chicken egg	3.1	3.8	1.4	423	1,148	74	15.51
tallow	49.8	41.8	4	109	3,100	600	5.17
pork fat	39.2	45.1	11.2	95	10,199	1,000	10.20
hazelnut	4.5	45.7	7.9		7,832	87	90.02
macadamia	12.1	58.9	1.5		1,296	206	6.29
pistachios	5.4	23.3	13.5		13,200	254	51.97
cashews	7.8	23.8	7.8		7,782	62	125.52
almonds	3.7	30.9	12.1		12,065	6	2010.83
walnuts	6.1	8.9	47.2		38,092	9,079	4.20
avocado	2.1	9.8	1.8		1,689	110	15.35

Legend:
SFA – saturated fatty acids g/100 g
MUFA – monounsaturated fatty acids g/100 g
PUFA – polyunsaturated fatty acids g/100 g
CH – cholesterol mg/100 g
O6 – omega-6 mg/100 g
O3 – omega-3 mg/100 g
O6:O3 – omega-6 to omega-3 ratio

Note: marks represent values that can depend on the type of particular food, location of its production and other environmental factors. The table was created for informative purposes – for accurate measurements, always check products individually.

MCT Oil

Now that you've looked at the table above and things are more or less clear to you. You may wonder what kind of genetically modified thing this MCT oil is, because this surely is something you don't want to put in your body.

Worry not: MCT oil is an extremely fine and useful thing. While the name may sound a bit technical, it is most commonly a mixture of coconut oil and oil from the kernels of African oil palm (*Elaeis guineensis*). You have to admit that it's simpler to say MCT, than a mixture of coconut oil and oil from the kernels of African oil palm! Apart from the name being more attractive, it also explains the magic behind this mixture: the oil that contains almost exclusively saturated medium-chain fatty acids (mainly caproic C6:0, caprylic C8:0 and capric C10:0 and tiny amounts of all other fatty acids).

Because you've thoroughly examined the table with the most important fatty acids, you now wonder what the difference between MCT oil and coconut oil is. There are two differences and although both irrelevant for recreational dieting enthusiasts, we will still mention them; MCT oil has a higher concentration of medium-chain fatty acids and – if it is good – less lauric acid (C12:0), which is known to have a slightly different effect on metabolism due to its length.

Medium-chain fatty acids get used directly for energy production and their metabolic process is substantially shorter compared to long-chain fatty acids. If you like to keep things easy, it is totally appropriate and correct to just use coconut oil.

So, what is the reason for giving oils full of medium-chain fatty acids their own chapter? These oils are distinct metabolic drivers; our bodies can easily and quickly use them for energy, they are transported to the brain using the shortest path and they are ketogenic which means they stimulate the production of ketone bodies. Because of their ketogenic nature, they often get used with disorders of absorption, malnutrition, and in diets of people with epilepsy. Studies also indicate they may be beneficial for Alzheimer's and Parkinson's disease.

Oils rich in medium-chain fatty acids are useful for the following reasons:

- by making us feel full, they help with our body composition, some studies show these fatty acids may work by increasing thermogenesis which can prevent fatty tissue from being formed;
- by beneficially affecting (and preventing) obesity, they lower risk factors for the development of the metabolic syndrome and consequently many other modern disease;
- they positively affect brain and gut and by doing so, they improve cognitive functions, well-being and energy levels;
- they have antibacterial, antiviral and antifungal effects;
- they don't require bile acids from the gall bladder for digestion therefore they enter the blood stream soon after consuming;
- because of their thermal stability and having no flavor and scent, they can be widely used for cooking.

Cholesterol

If you found the last chapter a bit too much, I kindly ask you to try and get through just these last few complicated facts that follow.

Cholesterol is a unique substance. It's a waxy substance which is so important for life that human body produces it itself – from saturated fatty acids. Cholesterol is formed in most cells, but predominantly in liver, gut and even in skin.

Healthy individuals produce 80 percent of all of their cholesterol by themselves and they consume the other 20 percent with food. By regulating the intake of cholesterol, we control only the small part of all combined body cholesterol.

Cholesterol is a component of cellular membrane: it enables cell fluidity and also plays a structural role, similar to the role of cellulose in plant cells. It is extremely significant for the synthesis of vitamin D and all steroid hormones (cortisol, aldosterone, progesterone, estrogen, testosterone and others), neurotransmission, proper functioning of serotonin receptors in the brain (low levels of cholesterol in blood are related to antisocial behavior and depression), healthy intestinal walls ...

You're probably shaking your head right now and thinking that cholesterol isn't just one substance, but at least two substances. Let's explain this unfortunate issue with its name. Cholesterol is indeed just one type of substance, carried through bloodstream by different types of protein. A combination of lipids (triglycerides, cholesterol, phospholipids) and the transporter (protein) is therefore called a lipoprotein. The names of individual lipoproteins indicate their chemical nature: cholesterol HDL (high-density lipoprotein) and cholesterol LDL (low-density lipoprotein). These two are most often talked about, but there are also three other large groups of lipoprotein: VLDL (very-low-density lipoprotein), IDL (intermediate density lipoprotein) and chylomicrons.

The density described in the names of these lipoproteins refers to the protein amount: cholesterol HDL has a higher share of protein and a lower share of fat, while on the other hand the VLDL has very little protein and is mostly composed of fats (cholesterol and triglycerides).

Because naming cholesterol based on individual transmitters has long been established, we've decided to also use it in this book: this means we speak of cholesterol HDL, cholesterol LDL etc.

You can imagine cholesterol being a worker, capable of doing certain jobs in a human body, while lipoprotein are little ships, transporting the worker to his workplace. What happens with cholesterol also depends on the type of transportation vessel it uses. The reason for that lies in the enemies waiting on its path capable of substantially damaging both the passenger and the vessel.

The HDL cholesterol is the good kind, or the protective cholesterol. It is some sort of an organism cleaner, which besides having functions in the cells, also takes care of the elimination of unused cholesterol from the arterial walls, preventing damage and clogging. Insufficient amounts of HDL cholesterol present a risk for development of cardiovascular disease, metabolic syndrome and even cancer.

The LDL cholesterol is known as the bad kind of cholesterol, but this isn't actually the case. Because vessels used for its transport are slower, they are more exposed to free radicals, the bad guys sent in by oxidative stress, which by oxidation break the vessel's engine and make it crash into arterial walls and cause damage. Another theory suggests that the LDL particles run aground on the walls of arteries, where they are meant to repair some of the damage caused by the free radicals, viruses and structural malfunctions. Regardless of the reasons making them run aground, the consequence is clear: when there are many of these vessels crashing, atherosclerosis develops.

One of the least known characteristics of the LDL cholesterol is the size difference of its particles – which is exactly what determines whether the LDL is the good or the bad kind. Smaller, more dense particles are more dangerous than the larger, fluffy kind. Some studies show that individuals with large amounts of LDL particles have far more chance of developing heart disease, whereas some hypotheses suggest that the large LDL particles could even be beneficial.

What does this actually mean? By bringing the size of the LDL particles into discussion, we debunk the belief that LDL is generally harmful. Research in recent years has shown that this statement is not completely true: the *small LDL particles* are harmful, while the large ones aren't (and may even be beneficial). Even if large LDL particles are actually beneficial, we're still having difficulties. Measuring the levels of LDL cholesterol poses a problem. The levels of LDL aren't *measured* using conventional methods, but are instead *calculated* based on a special formula, that subtracts the HDL cholesterol and part of the VLDL cholesterol, from total cholesterol (google the Friedewald equation, to learn more).

This means that when you get your blood results, they are *calculated* based on assumptions to present the LDL cholesterol amount. This piece of information only describes the total amount of LDL cholesterol and does not at all mention the number of LDL particles or their size. Theoretically, you could have very high LDL, but a small LDL particle count (meaning large size particles) – which would be good news.

Why is this so? Precise measurement of the amount and size of the LDL particles is more difficult, takes longer and costs more, therefore in routine check-ups you receive a calculated value of LDL cholesterol's mass, without any information on the size of the particles.

Despite all that, things aren't all bad. For the time being, it seems we can get a rough estimate of the amount of small and large LDL particles based upon triglyceride levels. The more triglycerides you have, the more of the small LDL particles there are and vice versa.

Cholesterol VLDL, a lipoprotein, mainly responsible for transportation of triglycerides, a bit less of cholesterol, has in recent years been proven to be very important. These "vessels" are small (small protein content), yet they carry a lot of passengers (fats) and are therefore even more likely to run aground on the arterial walls and according to the latest studies, are even more dangerous than the LDL cholesterol.

It is therefore worth remembering: small levels of HDL cholesterol are a bad sign, whereas high levels of LDL aren't necessarily a bad thing: they are only dangerous if the triglyceride level is also high.

Carbohydrate Restriction Diets

Unless you're one of those people, who test out every single diet that makes its way on the market, then you might be getting a bit confused with the names. These days, a lot can be heard about the paleo, *primal* diet, Dr. Atkins diet, LCHF, ketogenic diet.

All of these dietary regimens have one thing in common: consuming food as similar as possible to the food which humans consumed before the agricultural revolution.

The idea behind all of these dietary approaches is based on the principle, that humans are evolutionarily adapted to food consumed by the hunters and gatherers. 10,000 years is a long period of time, hard for us to imagine (it's 133 lifetimes, if each life is 75 years long), yet looking at it from the perspective of evolution, it is an extremely short period in which any significant adaption surely wasn't possible or probable.

Just think about it – humans have existed for 2 to 2.5 million years: if we ignore modern history, then we have basically survived this entire time from things we found in nature. If human history from Homo habilis onward was represented by the distance from US Mexican to US Canadian border, then humans began cultivating their food somewhere *around* Plentywood, Montana. That's how little time human history from agricultural revolution onward proportionally represents.

If you consumed nothing but game, wild berries and roots all the way through Texas, New Mexico, Colorado and Wyoming and started binging on mush, grits, porridge and bread in Plentywood, then further towards Canada you'd start stuffing yourself with more bread, pasta, noodles in the evening and finished it off with cakes and sugary soda like it was your last day and nothing mattered … then it could as well be your last day, as you'd suffer from swelling, pain, bloating and would be desperate to find the closest public toilet to spew your guts out by the time you approached the border.

This of course is just a guess.

No one really knows for sure whether we've already managed to adapt to different food in 10,000 years. The fact is there actually are a few studies indicating that – since we began eating grains and drinking domestic animals' milk, we've managed to adapt.

To a certain degree.

By studying the DNA found in human remains dating before the agricultural revolution and comparing it to the modern human DNA, the scientists have found *some* recent genetic adaptations, for example the salivary gene, responsible for digestion of starch and for fighting tooth decay caused by starch rich food, among others [6].

On the other hand, there is some proof that certain aspects of immunity existed before humans started to live as farmers – in close proximity to animals and in densely populated areas. In 2006, skeletons of two males were found at the La Braña-Arintero site in Spain, dating 7,000 year back, when Europe was not yet subjected to the Middle Eastern agricultural revolution. Based on genomic sequence of one of those two man, it was proven that some adaptive variants associated with pathogen resistance in modern Europeans were already present in this hunter-gatherer and did not occur during the adaptation to the farming lifestyle as was previously hypothesized [7].

The scientists have made no conclusions, while many agree that in the last 10,000 years, there were not enough adaptations to claim we have adapted to the changes in our dietary habits that were brought over with the Neolithic revolution. To put it shortly – despite some genetic adaptation – humans today are still more like the prehistoric humans and less like humans – farmers. Until we learn more, it remains a fact that Homo sapiens in its 40,000 years since crawling on the face of the Earth, has seen very few adaptations, very negligible when it comes to food based on farming and even less so, when it comes to processed food sold in supermarkets in recent decades.

It's still worth retaining some doubt whether we are like our prehistoric ancestors from a dietary perspective and what that could potentially mean. We cannot ignore the fact that when looked at from the evolutionary point of view, individual's health and life duration are almost completely insignificant: it's only important they live long enough to reproduce and ensure their offspring survive – if possible, long enough for offspring to breed.

Nowadays, we all feel like we are the center of our world and intend to live long, so this may come as a surprise: talking about genetic adaptations means talking about children who survived and had children of their own. Those are our ancestors who carry these potential adaptations. When it comes to menopausal women and grandpas doing 100 pull ups with ease before breakfast, the evolution fits in only to a degree: these people are more of a curiosity for anthropologists and those studying evolutionary peculiarities.

What does this mean?

If a human consumed arsenic but survived until their children were born, and they didn't die too soon, then this was considered and evolutionary success.

Of course no one actually consumed arsenic, but looking at modern humans, we can see that it's irrelevant if a person lives off cereal, cheeseburgers or a combination of ham, lettuce and nuts. The important bit is being able to have children who have a high chance of surviving. At 40 years of age, an individual like that could pass away and as far as evolution goes, it wouldn't be a loss of any kind. Life goes on. In this regard, the Neolithic revolution was a tremendous achievement: as there are 7 and a half billion people on Earth today, most fed by the food we, as a species only came by 10,000 years ago.

Could it also be – that we were in some aspects already adapted to the Neolithic diet and further adaptation wasn't necessary? What if disease and problems modern humans deal with appeared because we haven't adapted our diets and ourselves to the modern way of living?

There are plenty of dilemmas out there, but this doesn't mean that healthy life and longevity can't be achieved by considering things that might be beneficial to us. It seems that by studying human diet even before the Neolithic revolution can answer some of our questions.

This kind of concept presents the grounds for the dietary regimens mentioned at the beginning of chapter, although there are some, mainly interpretative differences between them. The grounds of the Paleo diet for instance, are based on the assumption that grass – no, not cannabis (cannabis actually isn't a type of grass) – but the modern types, we call grain, along with enticing product of sugarcane, are the reason for everything bad in our diet. The Paleo movement has grown in the last 30 years, ever since in 1985 Boyd Eaton and Melvin Konner published a paper in the New England Journal of Medicine, mostly addressing the problems of grain consumption [8].

The proponents of the Paleo and primal diet claim there are two main problems with grain: gluten, a protein found in grain, meant to cause all sorts of issues, and indigestible bran, which might cause microdamage inside the human gut, leading to chronic inflammatory conditions, or even poisoning.

Then there's a group of related dietary regimens that include LCHF, Dr. Atkins diet and ketogenic diet. These are like the two mentioned before, but with less ideology attached to them and looking more promising from a scientific point of view. All three are based on general acknowledgment of harmful effects of a high carbohydrate intake. The grounds for these claims come from discoveries about human metabolic processes – which we more than likely brought through to modern times from the period before the Neolithic revolution.

This book introduces the theoretical and practical aspects of ketogenic diet and its variations. As we will soon reveal, the secret of this diet lies in the dietary ketosis, also known as physiological ketosis. The LCHF is a variation of ketogenic diet that involves a bit more carbohydrates, mostly from vegetables, nuts and occasionally some chocolate.

★ *By the way: a low carbohydrate intake diet was mentioned for the first time back in the 1863, when an English undertaker William Banting published the Letter on corpulence, addressed to the public (a letter about obesity addressed to the public) [9]. The booklet was so popular that a part of his surname became a synonym for a low carbohydrate intake diet and dieting in general: do you bant? William Banting was*

Dr. Atkins Diet

Some of you readers are already very familiar with the diet of Dr. Atkins, a renowned cardiologist who published his first version of the diet in the early 70s and later in life revised it several times (the first version of his diet was very similar to the standard ketogenic diet). Atkins' dietary plan is – like the ketogenic and the LCHF diets – focused on carbohydrate restriction in a diet. Although it emphasizes on the importance of fat consumption, it differs from the ketogenic diet in this exact detail, since Atkins diet requires quite a lot of protein intake, whereas fats are consumed a bit less substantially. In this regard, the Atkins diet is more like the LCHF, although they are not quite the same.

One of the most interesting points of the modified Atkins diet is also useful for all of you willing to give the ketogenic diet a go. The Atkins diet namely consists of different phases:

• in the first so-called induction phase that should last around two weeks, the individual restricts carbohydrate intake to less than 20 grams per day and obtains those mainly from vegetables. The difference when compared to the ketogenic diet is the recommended protein and fat intake, while the carbohydrate restriction is the same and has similar effects as the first stage of the ketogenic diet;

• in the second, so-called balancing phase, in which the individual stays until they weigh roughly 10 pounds more than their target weight, more vegetables, berries, nuts and seeds are added to the diet – while the daily carbohydrate intake goes up to 50 g;

• in the third, so-called pre-maintenance phase, the individual gradually starts increasing the carbohydrate intake by 10 grams per day and monitoring their body weight, determining the ideal amount of consumed carbohydrates that still allows them to lose weight. Ideally this amounts to 50 and 80 g;

• the last phase is the maintenance phase and represents the new dietary habits we've learned in the previous three phases. In the third phase, each individuals is able to define the limit amount of carbohydrates consumed daily, that's still allowing them to lose and not gain weight. In the maintenance phase, they stick to the set limit. Newly acquired habits help individuals to maintain their body weight and ensure they don't bail and return to their previous diet and fat accumulation.

What is the Ketogenic Diet and How Does It Work

To keep it short and simple: the ketogenic diet is a dietary approach that involves a substantial intake of dietary fats, less of protein and very little of carbohydrates. When most of our energy comes from the consumed fats, we experience dietary ketosis, a crucial factor for a number of beneficial effects, which this type of dieting has on our body.

Dietary Ketosis – When Blood Glucose Levels Drop
Despite the fact that our body finds it easier to get energy from glucose, it can – as seen in the previous chapter – also get energy from fats. Those are broken down into fatty acids through a complex metabolic process and

used for energy and other functions. When fatty acids are used or processed in the liver, ketone bodies begin forming. Ketones are also produced when consuming carbohydrates, but the quantities of ketone bodies are much smaller.

Conditions that make our body produce substantial amounts of ketone bodies can be achieved through three different ways, all of which are characterized by decreased insulin levels.

These three ways are:

• starving (not recommended unless we're talking about a planned a carefully structured fast or the intermittent fasting, both can actually be very beneficial),

• low insulin levels (recommended, unless accompanied by high levels of glucose that is caused by type 1 diabetes which lowers levels of insulin) and

• manipulating blood glucose levels with a diet rich in dietary fats, very little protein and almost no carbohydrates.

Insulin can be quite troublesome, which we'll describe later, because there's a special condition occurring in diabetes patients that is responsible for giving ketone bodies and dietary ketosis a bad name.

Let's stick with healthy people for now. Let's say there's a student name Mark, who ran out of bread, pasta, sweets and fruit, but has a large supply of sausages and butter at home. To prevent the food from going to waste, Mark decides that during his studies for exams, he will use the supply he has available.

After a few meals consisting from pieces of sausage decorated with buttery swirls, the glucose levels in his blood drop. Insulin, which reacts to the presence of glucose like a dog when you open the refrigerator door, is left idle, therefore the levels of insulin remain low and steady. Mark's organism begins using the consumed fats (and if needed, also his body fat), while at the same time the liver begin producing ketone bodies when processing these fats.

Mark is a healthy individual and his liver is able to produce up to 185 grams of ketones daily. The body knows that these ketone bodies are useful and begins sending them out to the type of tissues that are capable of using them as a valuable energy source.

Because Mark continues to eat fat only, there are plenty of ketone bodies being produced – more than the body can effectively use. After a few days, Mark's heart and muscles become increasingly more efficient at using fatty acids, while the ketone bodies get used only by those organs, which can't convert free fatty acids into energy – for instance, the brain, which tends to be quite over-loaded because of Mark's exam period. During these days of adaptation, the production of ketones also settles and the organism starts to adapt to a high-fat diet.

Mark is now in a dietary ketosis and gets to enjoy all of the benefits this type of condition brings, most of all, the constantly low levels of insulin, less oxidative stress, and, consequently, less inflammation.

Dietary ketosis is a condition with increased levels of ketone bodies while the glucose and insulin levels remain stable. It occurs when a body begins using mostly consumed fats or body fat as energy, because there isn't enough glucose in the blood. During metabolic processing of these fats, the liver starts forming ketone bodies (this is called ketogenesis), which also get used as energy.

Formation of ketone bodies is a completely natural process in healthy individuals, allowing the body to adapt to food shortages, or more specifically, to the shortage of glucose.

Healthy people are able to regulate metabolism and have proportionate levels of insulin, glucagon, epinephrine and other metabolic hormones, therefore blood sugar for them isn't a problem. Low levels of insulin, normal levels of glucagon and epinephrine, along with low levels of blood sugar, cause a release of fatty acids from fat tissue. These fatty acids travel to liver, where they are transformed into ketone bodies.

These bodies then re-enter the bloodstream and the body uses them as energy.

These processes happen whenever we don't eat (enough) for a certain period of time: early in the morning, during restrictive dieting, long activities and during starvation.

Ketogenic Spectrum: Dietary Ketosis is Different to Ketoacidosis

Let's head back and look at the reasons why the ketogenic diet is often given a bad name. Simply put: it is because of a lack of understanding of the difference between dietary ketosis and diabetic ketoacidosis. Ketoacidosis, or diabetic ketoacidosis, is a deadly condition mostly affecting diabetics, whereas dietary ketosis is just a body's natural response to lower levels of glucose in our blood.

As we shall see later, both of these conditions are parts of a similar process, yet only one of them is considered to be normal and beneficial. We can compare this to music: when listening to music at a normal volume, we are able to enjoy it and even experience a positive physiological response, but when turning the volume on full blast, this same type of music can suddenly cause excruciating pain, suffering and even inflict irreparable injuries upon our body.

The source of all major issues in diabetic patients lies in insulin, a hormone regulating the blood glucose levels in a healthy human body: it is responsible for distributing glucose to the cells, where it gets used as energy, or in cases where there is too much glucose in the blood, the storing of it in the form of fat tissue. To prevent excessive levels of glucose, insulin also has the ability to regulate gluconeogenesis.

In patients with diabetes insulin does not function well. Type 1 diabetes appears when the insulin producing cells in the pancreas completely deteriorate, resulting in insufficient insulin levels. The cause of this is yet to be determined. Type 2 diabetes is, on the other hand, mostly a result of a developed condition. Due to constant excessive insulin levels, the cells protect themselves by becoming less sensitive to insulin – this stage of prediabetes is known as the insulin resistance, or the resistance of cells to insulin. It is followed by an even greater production of insulin, which the human body finds increasingly harder to use and which can lead to a drastic decline in insulin production and to glucose metabolism disorders.

The consequences of insulin related problems are, in both of these cases, possible toxic blood glucose levels and the inability of the body to regulate and lower the excessive amount of glucose.

To put it simply, this means that the body, despite having too much glucose in its blood, thinks it has no useful energy available and starts using fat to function. As we have seen earlier, ketone bodies are formed during metabolism of fats and when there are enough of them we get into state of ketosis. No problems appear if the body is in dietary ketosis and levels of insulin and glucose remain normal.

But in individuals with diabetes, things usually aren't as smooth; they can have abnormally high levels of glucose AND at the same time high levels of ketones in their blood. This is no longer a ketosis, but a ketoacidosis, which can be lethal. Diabetic ketoacidosis presents realistic danger for type 1 diabetics, alcoholics and people with certain other medical conditions (ketotic hypoglycemia in children, insufficient amounts of growth hormone, alcohol poisoning and some other rare dysfunctions of lipid and ketone body metabolism).

To be honest, dietary ketosis and ketoacidosis are both related conditions stretching over a spectrum. However, they differ in three parameters:

- in the blood, levels of ketone bodies during dietary ketosis is between 0.5 to 4.0 mmol/l[1], after a few days of fasting from 4 to 7, whereas with ketoacidosis the ketone levels rise above 10 mmol/l and even higher (as high as 20);
- in glucose levels: in dietary ketosis, glucose levels remain low, or stable and in ketoacidosis they are too high;
- During ketoacidosis blood pH is low. In dietary ketosis pH remains normal.

---

[1] There are different estimations of what range of ketone bodies' concentration represents the dietary ketosis. Even the concentration of 7.0 mmol/l can still be an effect of dietary induced ketosis. On top of that, different ketones' concentrations have different strength of effect: sometimes a migraine sufferer will be headache free in the lower ranges of dietary ketosis, while appetite suppression in order to lose weight will require higher concentrations of ketones. Biological individuality also plays a role – so it is important to know that 3.0 mmol/l will do A for person AA, but might have the effect B for the person BB.

A small amount of ketone bodies are constantly present in our body even of we consume carbohydrates. In normal conditions their levels are low – up to 0.2 mmol/l, or in certain circumstances slightly more (obesity, physical activity, meal arrangement, diabetes).

Levels of ketone bodies in blood of healthy people on an average diet are usually the highest in the morning, when we can measure levels up to 0.5 mmol/l, whereas more normal values are between 0.1 and 0.2 mmol/l. These quantities are barely perceivable using the measuring methods.

If we are starving or if we lower the intake of carbohydrates, the production of ketone bodies in liver will gradually increase and with that their blood levels. When healthy individuals are in dietary ketosis, the levels can be increased as much as 10 times of the normal value. At the same time their insulin and glucose levels remain low or stable.

An optimal interval for blood levels of ketone bodies in dietary ketosis is subject to interpretation: some speak of values between 0.5 and 3.0 mmol/l, but this can also be higher. If increased levels of ketone bodies occur simultaneously with high levels of glucose, diabetic ketoacidosis is likely the problem, for example levels of ketone bodies can be as high as 40 mmol/l.

A diet with a normal intake of carbohydrates	from less than 0.1 to 0.3 mmol/l
A diet with a very limited intake of carbohydrates	from 0.5 to 5.0 mmol/l
Fasting/starvation (at least a week)	5.0 to 7.0 mmol/l
Ketoacidosis	10 to 20 and more mmol/l

Dietary ketosis is a metabolic process, whereas ketoacidosis is a dangerous disorder which can occur with type 1 diabetes and also with extreme alcohol abuse. Ketoacidosis, although rare, is also possible in type 2 diabetes patients.

Measuring Levels of Ketone Bodies

As we've seen, dietary ketosis is no bogeyman like many who don't understand it is different to ketoacidosis, still believe.

In the process of ketogenesis, with lower blood glucose levels, the liver starts forming ketone bodies, which include acetone, acetoacetate and beta-hydroxybutyrate. When ketogenic diets are used as a form of therapy such as with athletes who use ketogenic diet to improve their athletic abilities, the exact levels of ketones is important information, therefore it is wise to measure them precisely.

For most healthy individuals, who are using ketogenic diet for weight loss, well-being and achieving mental agility, measuring in most cases isn't necessary. It can be useful in the initial phase of self evaluation, the measurements can also be considered as a source of motivation.

We can find the optimal intake levels of carbohydrates using the observation method. It is worth knowing that the ketone levels and the amount of weight we lose aren't directly related. Some will feel the effects of the ketogenic diet even with relatively low levels of ketogenic ketone bodies, whereas others will require higher levels.

We can measure the levels of ketone bodies using three different methods. Each method has different accessibility and reliability in determining the degree of dietary ketosis.

Through Urine

The ketone levels in urine are measured using special strips that indicate the level of acetoacetate. Unfortunately this piece of information is pretty useless for determining the current state of dietary ketosis, since it shows only the amount of excess ketones we eliminated through urine. Another problem is that acetoacetate is only detectable in urine during initial phases, or when transitioning to ketosis, while later the body can reabsorb acetoacetate and at the same time adjust its production according to needs, so there are no excess amounts and it therefore can't be detected in urine. The more an individual is adapted to ketone utilization the less ketones there are in urine. The measured levels of ketone bodies also depend on hydration: the more we are hydrated, the lower the levels of ketone bodies will appear, although this can be deceiving. By measuring acetoacetate we can get low levels reading and can inaccurately assume we aren't in dietary ketosis.

Through Exhaled Air

We measure ketone levels in exhaled air using analyzers of exhaled air using a device quite similar to police breathalyzers.

We measure the amount of acetone in the exhaled air, but just like with levels of ketone bodies measured in urine, this piece of data is only partially reliable, since the obtained results are from intervals and are not accurately expressed with mmol/l.

The levels of acetone in exhaled air are an indicator of whether the body is in dietary ketosis, but they don't tell us much about the amount of beta-hydroxybutyrate in blood. Acetone in exhaled air will appear soon after we cease with carbohydrate consumption, its amount will remain stable, as long as there are still glycogen reserves present in the body. Once those are depleted, the amount of exhaled acetone also increases.

Analyzing exhaled air can also help determine individual's sensitivity to certain foods, or with monitoring the effects of particular foods on the overall amount of ketone bodies in an organism. Since measuring ketosis via exhaled air is relatively inexpensive, it can be checked more frequently and can help establish patterns of the individual's response to the macronutrient intake.

Through Blood

By measuring blood levels of ketone bodies, we measure levels of beta-hydroxybutyrate. This type of measuring is reliable, accurate and most useful for establishing the stage of dietary ketosis we are in. Measuring beta-hydroxybutyrate is reasonable, if we haven't been consuming carbohydrates for some time, since the amount of these ketone bodies gradually grows during the adaptation period to a fat rich diet. Also, since this ketone body decreases during the exercise due to energy uptake, it should not be measured directly afterwards.

Unfortunately, this method is expensive, invasive and quite inaccessible to regular population. It's reasonable if you use the ketogenic diet due to medical issues or if you're a professional athlete. The rest of us can learn how to observe dietary ketosis through different effects intake of foods have on us.

Criticism of the Ketogenic Diet

It would most definitely be easier to list all possible beneficial effects of the ketogenic diet, if the production, food processing or pharmaceutical industries could sell it. Like with every other novelty it's worth asking "who does this benefit", but sometimes it is OK to instead ask "who does NOT benefit from this".

There are no doubt a lot of people with profound dietary knowledge among the critics of the ketogenic diet, who think that the ketogenic diet and its effects, especially long-term ones, have not been researched meticulously enough to be considered acceptable. This is a totally relevant consideration, we do want to keep alive throughout this entire book. Also, imagine if you were a respected dietary expert, who's been explaining and advising on nutrition your whole career and using one of the dietary pyramids as your basis and advising against (excessive and/or saturated) fat consumption. How do you then suddenly say, hey, sorry, but last 15 years have shown that this persecution of fat and worshiping anything that grows in a grain field may not be as great as it seemed?

Aversion to ketogenic diet will definitely be present among the cynics on duty, who are most commonly people who have never experienced any dietary problems, or dealt with the consequences of dietary problems. These are the people who never seem to accumulate any fat, or if that does happen, they can just throw a glimpse at running shoes, adapt their diet a little *et voilà* – they're back in excellent shape. They often advocate moderation and lots of exercise in order to achieve goals, which for them come in form of a fairly pimped out body structure and sharply carved out six pack muscles looking like a lethal weapon. But even the cynics have good reasons to be skeptical: they are sick of all kinds of dietary fabrications, flooding the public space that only work due to constant dietary restrictions, while people forget that the results of these diets should be more apparent. To sum it up, a bunch of deceitful and spectacular sounding diets based on no solid ground whatsoever, work by convincing us of existing shortcuts, then let us down, when we find ourselves in the middle of a dark forest after sunset.

Criticism and skepticism is always worth considering – not just with dieting, but in life in general. Without criticism and skepticism anything can become religion – although without priests in Halloween costumes. However, if we're not allowed to raise doubts over dogmas, then we're sorry, this just isn't it.

If we ignore the categorical nihilists, people who spend decades building their reputation based on low fat hysteria and cynics, the criticism of the ketogenic diet is often based on the following arguments:

*   high-fat diets are hard to stick with and maintain in the long run;
*   high-fat diets cause constipation and harm gut flora;
*   high-fat diets cause insulin resistance in cells;
*   high-fat diets present a good environment for developing inflammatory conditions. ;
*   high-fat diets cause vitamin and mineral deficiency; vitamin C deficiency in particular, which can lead to scurvy;
*   weight loss on a high-fat diet is the result of losing body fluids, not body fat;
*   high-fat diets can cause thyroid issues, mainly an insufficient production of thyroid hormones;
*   high fat diets increase levels of blood lipids, mainly LDL cholesterol;
*   high-fat diets cause kidney stones;
*   high-fat diets aren't suitable for top level athletes
*   and because high-fat diets aren't suitable for top level athletes, they're not suitable for anyone.

If you're considering the ketogenic diet, you shouldn't take any of these ideas lightly (except the last one). Use them to help you focus on what's important. Constipation, vitamin and mineral deficiency, potential harmful changes in blood count ... all of these can be monitored. In fact it is recommended you do so, if you decide to make such drastic changes to your diet. There are no real compelling scientific grounds for most of these arguments. On the contrary, the scientific studies that do exist indicate the opposite, as we will later show in the chapter *(Therapeutic) Effects of the Ketogenic Diet.*

Many may encounter difficulties sticking with a high-fat diet. The reasons vary. Maybe you're unhappy with the choice of foods because you love fruit so much. Maybe you'll struggle to stick with the diet because of your friends and family. Maybe you travel a lot and simply don't have the time to eat high-fat meals exclusively. Maybe you'll get bored of all the good things. All of this is true – but it is in no way specific to the ketogenic diet.

Persisting with something that restricts us in one way or another is usually hard to do. This is particularly true for diets with a restrictive energy intake. This is exactly the reason behind the popularity of the ketogenic diet. It is the only kind that, without a prior restriction of energy intake, can lead over time to a lower energy intake without making you feel deprived or needing to exert excessive self-restraint. Not only that, but many report that they experience a shift in their dietary preferences. If they get to choose between pizza and heavily buttered eggs, they would rather feast upon the latter.

When applying ketogenic diets to athletes, things are a bit more specific, although we shouldn't understand this as a potential theory suggesting the diet isn't suitable for them.

Can You Assure That the Ketogenic Diet Isn't Just a Trend?

We can't. However, this book is the result of the enthusiasm of satisfied users and researchers into its benefits. In an educational and fun science paper about dietary approaches and diabetes control, written by British dietitians Lyn Sawyer and Edwin Gale, they state that, sadly, "passion in science is an infallible marker of lack of evidence" [10]. Therefore the purpose of this book isn't to make you blindly believe in every word we say (we'd rather not abuse the blind but help them, thanks).

But until someone comes up with a chemical substance in the form of a pill that will make users slim, healthy, mentally agile and enable them live longer, the ketogenic diet can't be considered as just a trend. A pill like that would be extremely awesome, we agree.

Another legitimate question is, how do we know that promoting the ketogenic diet isn't just a joke, as proved to be the case with Ancel Keys' studies of the dangers of fat consumption? Doubt is understandable – if we as a society got tricked once, we don't want to let ourselves fall for it again. However, this shouldn't be the reason for not believing in science and scientific methods. Quite the contrary. Science can be wrong, but it must admit its mistakes. Sooner or later.

(Therapeutic) Effects of the Ketogenic Diet

Despite being used today as a method for improving body composition, or weight loss as it's usually referred to, the ketogenic diet derives from medicine. Greek doctors have long been familiar with the benefits of fasting for patients with epilepsy. In the 1920s the diet was introduced as a suitable alternative to the starving of patients with epilepsy. It wasn't until the 1960s that it also became known as a weight loss diet.

Intentionally induced dietary ketosis also has other kinds of therapeutic potential. Very early on it was also used as a diet in the treatment of diabetes – one of the first documented examples of successfully controlling diabetes with the ketogenic diet dates back to 1899. Doctor Elliot Joslin's mother spent 14 years on a diet consisting of approximately 40-70 grams of carbohydrates and 150 grams of fats per day.

It also seems that fat consumption, presuming the carbohydrate intake is low, doesn't present any danger regarding the development of cardiovascular disease, but instead has a beneficial – opposite – effect.

The ketogenic diet produces quite convincing results in epilepsy, weight loss and cardiovascular disease, while there are still studies being carried out into the connections between the ketogenic diet and its therapeutic effects on irritable bowel syndrome, gastroesophageal reflux, migraine, chronic pain, cancer, polycystic ovary syndrome, neurological diseases such as Alzheimer's and Parkinson's, brain damage and Lou Gehrig's disease (ALS) and even acne. The list of hypothetical ideas is long, but we'd like stick with those mentioned in order to avoid allegations of scandalous speculation.

Overweight and Obesity

Acknowledging modern society's obesity problem probably doesn't need special arguments to back it up (although we've already done that – see the chapter *How Did we Manage to Get So Fat?*).

While it is true that society today lacks the sense for appropriate self-assessment and we consequently see numerous masochistic approaches to transforming our bodies, there's still a large proportion of us who actually are overweight, even if we don't count those who have no problems with the question of their bodies' looks.

Countless years of public health policies, the public emergence of a weight loss concept and constant individual efforts to achieve a more balanced body composition – all these phenomena evidently have the opposite effect to what is desired. Dietary and fitness recommendations don't help, neither do "weight loss" medications, and bariatric surgery is only suitable for clinically obese individuals (body mass index of at least 29).

Instead of becoming slimmer, more agile and ready to live a long life, we're heading in a totally wrong direction. Not only are we not pleased with ourselves, but by being overweight we make ourselves susceptible to a range of diseases that could easily be avoided. We're still unable to predict or prevent numerous diseases. Most of those which are prevalent today, such as type 2 diabetes, high blood pressure, cardiovascular disease and even certain types of cancer, begin with excessive nutrition and obesity.

A common belief is that obesity starts in the kitchen (and in the basement where those running shoes are accumulating dust in the back of a drawer) and after all these years we are still left without a clear and straight answer to the questions of what to do, how and what precisely to eat and how much we should exercise in order to lose weight. There actually are a few useful answers to those questions, but they are difficult to comply with and today's society dislikes and tends to avoid anything involving the word "difficult".

This accusation isn't based on us being childish and impatient by wanting immediate results with no effort (even though we're not immune to that either). Western society lifestyles, especially in the last 20 years, have become remarkably fast. By fast, we're talking about a drastic increase in the number of decisions we're required to make in every given moment – this can doubtlessly be attributed in large part to modern communication technologies.

From a physiological point of view the decision making process is extremely energy demanding. It's based on glucose consumption and it's no surprise that when mentally drained, you crave sweet things. This is called decision fatigue and can lead to a number of wrong decisions in life. Including being unable to stick with the diet that, only last Monday, you claimed was the ultimate weapon which would finally allow you to say goodbye to your body fat deposits.

The inner strength to persist with things we find demanding and which require self-control from us is a similar phenomenon. Once we implement self-control in too many areas of our lives, a condition occurs which psychologists call ego depletion.

Decision fatigue and ego depletion make us vulnerable to environmental temptations, including TV ads full of tasty looking food, shelves full of sweets right in your line of sight at the supermarket cashier, and of course the supplies of food at home, which wouldn't be a problem if it was eaten in moderation.

What use is the doctor's advice to eat a bit of everything – but in a moderate amount? What matters in every kind of therapeutic approach are two things: the desired results and that the process is bearable and survivable. We know how to kill off cancer cells in a petri dish, the problem is killing cancer cells of a living body. If the therapy is in any way painful, uncomfortable, impractical, the patient might become hesitant to cooperate. The World Health Organization (WHO) estimates that the average compliance with doctors' advice in patients suffering from chronic disease is at a mere 50 percent [11].

There are numerous compliance factors related to weight loss programs: from the price of foods of the particular regimen, individual taste and preference, personality structure, motivation and so on. Unfortunately, no irrefutable statistical proof exists that would show which dietary regimen is the easiest to maintain long-term (although there have been attempts towards finding it [12]), but based on the evident failure of the recommendations so far, we can only speculate that we need a more efficient and less tiring methods for improving body composition. At this point we can only rely on anecdotal evidence (and promising but modest scientific literature): many find the ketogenic diet to be extremely suitable.

Popularity of the Ketogenic Diet Among Users
Why are ketogenic diets so popular among people who are trying to lose weight? Easily put, the combine user experience speaks of a number of psycho-physiological effects (which affect compliance with the prescribed diet and consequently help with achieving the desired effects). Most experience:
- drastically decreased appetite;
- drastically decreased need to think about food;
- drastically lower sense of being restricted and because of it lower need for self control;
- increased sense of focus and mental power (the lack of both is a common problem and the reason to bail with other restrictive diets).

The mechanisms of the ketogenic diet, which the individual doesn't experience directly are:
- lowered lipogenesis and increased lipolysis (formation and decomposition of fat cells);
- higher oxygen consumption during fat metabolism (compared to glucose metabolism);
- formation of glucose through gluconeogenesis, a high energy-consuming process. It's estimated that an average person needs between 60-65 grams of glucose

per day – unless obtained with food, it is formed through gluconeogenesis of protein, or glycerol. In a study published in 2009, it was measured that the process of glucose formation equals 33 percent of the energy value of the glucose, while almost half of the increase of the basal metabolic rate is down to gluconeogenesis [13];

• in individuals who have already developed insulin resistance in cells, the glucose tolerance improves. Disturbance of glucose tolerance can result in increased lipogenesis (formation of fat out of glucose which the body is unable to use). Once these issues are resolved this can further contribute to weight loss, or a decrease of the amount of body fat tissue.

Lowered Appetite and Hunger During the Ketogenic Diet

A few hypotheses exist, but the exact mechanism of the effects the ketogenic diet has on lowering appetite is yet to be established. It could be that the appetite is directly affected by ketone bodies. One of the hypothesis claims that the appetite is lower due to stable glucose levels and consequently insulin. Dietary ketosis can effect in a lower appetite by secretion of cholecystokinin, AMP activated protein-kinase, gamma-aminobutyric acid and adiponectin [14].

Lower appetite affects an individual in two ways that both contribute them in achieving set goals: in most cases the daily energy intake automatically gets lower, while it also makes it easier to stick with the diet. This way the user falls into a positive cycle: the diet is easy to stick with, their body weight is dropping, motivation is maintained, an individual carries on.

Science on Obesity and the Ketogenic Diet

If you do a search for the words "*ketone*" and "*obesity*" in the Pubmed scientific literature database, it becomes clear that the interest of science in options offered by the ketogenic diet for battling obesity and overnutrition, is huge.

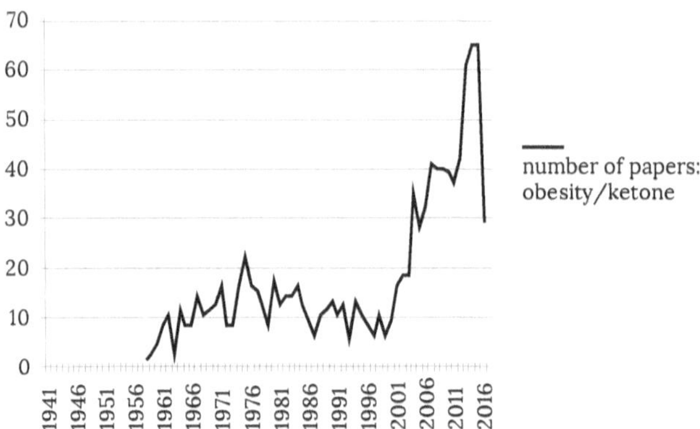

The graph above[2] shows the interest in the ketone ratio (or ketogenic diet) and *obesity in* the last 60 years. It is especially important to notice the dramatic increase of interest in the correlation between these two phenomena in the last 15 years.

A lot of published results doesn't necessarily mean that the ketogenic diet is definitely helping against obesity, but it's a good indication that the researchers found something that could potentially shift the paradigm which claims the best way to lose weight and balance body composition, is to avoid consuming fat.

Just for a laugh, let's try analyzing the number of results "*obesity*" and "*dietary fat*".

---

2   The graph and the following three similar graphs were created with the information gained through the free tool called Medsum (http://webtools.mf.uni-lj. si/public/medsum.html)

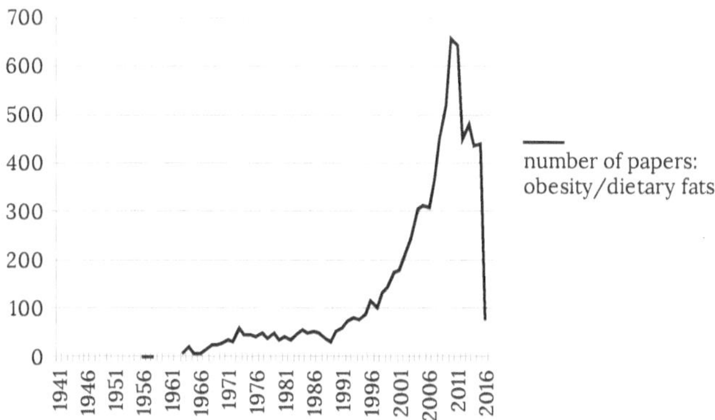

This graph also clearly shows a drastic increase of interest in the correlation of obesity and dietary fats in the last 15 years. It is also evident that the total number of these studies is far larger than that of studies that include the keywords ketone and obesity. As with the previous graph, it is again worth mentioning that the graph doesn't demonstrate any content relation of obesity and dietary fats, it only shows the drastic increase in the amount of publications that include these two key words. This brings us to conclude that scientists are interested in these topics and we can safely assume, are making sure that unlike Dr. Ancel Keys and his anti-fat crusade, we are not mistaken and supported with poor science. So, have we been misled by "anti-fatters"? We don't know, but for now it seems we've been.

The latest study, published just as this book was being created comes from Rome. It was a randomized clinical trial, examining effectiveness of two types of dietary approach: the ketogenic diet with a very low carbohydrate intake along with amino acidic supplement and a very energy restrictive diet. They were examining 25 healthy people. They concluded that the ketogenic diet is effective in weight loss and it also doesn't not lower person's muscle mass [15].

Similar conclusions were made by their colleagues near Naples, lead by Dr. Guiseppe Castaldo, who in 2016 published results of a study involving 73 obese people who took part in a two-phase weight loss program: three weeks of ketogenic diet followed by 6 weeks of hypocaloric diet on food with a low glycemic index, very similar to the Mediterranean diet. Both phases showed an improvement in belly fat, liver enzymes, levels of the growth hormone, blood pressure and metabolism of glucose and fat. It is interesting that many participants experienced an increase in levels of blood lipids and worse glucose tolerance in the phase involving the Mediterranean-like diet. Participants, already diagnosed with metabolic syndrome before taking part in the study and who generally got better results in the program, didn't experience this sort of decline. Based on this, the researchers conclude that cycling of the ketogenic and Mediterranean diet is especially suitable for people with the metabolic syndrome [16].

Another group of researchers, again lead by Dr. Castaldo, also tested the ketogenic diet on morbidly obese patients. A group of 112 patients were fed enteral nutrition without carbohydrates, through the nasogastric tube, followed by 14 days of orally consuming food with identical macro nutritional value. After a month they established that the effects of both types of feeding were identical: statistically significant lower body mass index, smaller waist circumference, lower blood pressure and an improved cell tolerance to insulin. Some of the participants have had their decrease of belly fat measured using an ultrasound. An increased amount of ketones did not affect kidney function or coagulation parameters. In a month long period they didn't witness any potential dangers of consuming food with no carbohydrate content [17].

Spanish researchers last year also published results of a study of the effects of adding the DHA polyunsaturated fatty acids in the diet of people prescribed to ketogenic diet. 29 overweight participants were placed into two groups and for a period of six months, both of them were using the ketogenic diet, but the DHA were added to just one of them. In the group that was receiving added DHA fatty acids they found a bunch of beneficial effects, mostly related to levels of anti-inflammatory response. Even more interesting is the fact that in six months the participants from both of the groups lost approximately 44 lbs of body weight (without any statistically significant differences between both groups) per average and that in the six months on the ketogenic diet, numerous biological indicators showed statistically significant improvements: glucose and insulin levels, triglycerides, LDL cholesterol, leptin and biomarkers connected with inflammatory response of a C-reactive protein, resistin (a.k.a. adipose tissue-specific secretory factor) and TNF-α – tumor necrosis factor alpha [18].

A different group of Spanish researchers from Madrid in 2014 published their results of a study in the Endocrine magazine, which was carried out on 79 people, suffering from overnutrition, split into two groups. One was using the principles of the ketogenic diet, while the other was using an energy restriction menu. Both groups were monitored for 12 months, they were given advice and were offered assistance with exercise etc. After 12 months, the members of the group using the ketogenic diet lost approximately 44 lbs of body weight, while the group with the restricted energy intake lost just 15 lbs. More than 88 percent individuals from the ketogenic group lost more than 10 percent of their initial bodyweight. In the group using the hypocaloric diet this was achieved by just 35 percent of individuals [19].

Systematic review of existing literature and meta analysis performed by Brazilian scientists, who analyzed 13 randomized clinical studies, brought similar conclusions. They combined the results of the studies that had to be randomized clinical studies, had to be at least 12 months in duration and compared the effects of the ketogenic and low-fat diet on adults. The ketogenic diet consisted of a daily intake of less than 50 grams of carbohydrates, whereas the low-fat diet got less than 30 percent of daily energy from fat).

What were the results? The test subjects using the ketogenic diet lost a statistically significant amount of body weight compared to the subjects on the low-fat diet. At the end of the study the ketogenic diet users also had significantly lower levels of blood triglycerides and lower diastolic blood pressure and increased HDL cholesterol. The levels of LDL cholesterol also increased (no data about the number or the size of particles). No statistically significant differences were found in systolic blood pressure, glucose and insulin levels when fasted, glycated hemoglobin A1c and C-reactive protein [20].

What's the Deal with Insulin?
Most people relate insulin to diabetes – surely you know someone with a genetic form of diabetes. People with type 1 diabetes need to regularly inject this important hormone. The majority of us lucky ones don't have to do that and only deal with insulin when some real clever book about dieting constantly tries drag it out of our gut (or our pancreas, to be precise), or when we are told we have type 2 diabetes, which is often connected with ignoring the wisdom found in clever books on dieting.

So what's so important about insulin that makes even healthy individuals know about its function?

To cut a long story short: insulin is a hormone that regulates metabolism. It's not the only one and it's often totally confused and confused insulin is a recipe for all sorts of trouble.

Confused insulin is like a grandma driving down the motorway in the wrong direction. It may just scare other drivers driving correctly, but it's more than likely going to cause a serious multiple-vehicle collision with everyone involved.

By using a less brief explanation, we can say that insulin is a hormone predominantly regulating what happens with consumed carbohydrates (also protein and fats, but to a substantially smaller degree), while it at the same time serves as a key for locking and unlocking individual's fat deposits. Therefore, if you are having trouble with excess body fat, it's worth knowing how to make insulin cooperate with you and help you get rid of the chunky fat bits.

Insulin is produced by the pancreas, a corncob like gland, positioned behind the stomach which has many other functions besides producing insulin. As we've mentioned earlier, insulin jumps whenever it senses high glucose levels, after eating a piece of bread or cake, a plate of pasta, or a tasty sandwich (the list is infinite, but to prevent you from drooling over things that make things tough for insulin, let's stick to that).

Once the blood glucose levels rise, insulin goes after it and begins distributing it to the cells, so they could use it as energy. Not only is it capable of distributing glucose to the cells, it can also persuade them to open up and use glucose. Without insulin we would basically die, since soon after a meal we'd have a fluid running through our veins, more similar to syrup or thin jam, than blood. We don't know about you, but to us that doesn't sound appealing.

Insulin keeps working for as long as the blood is too sweet. It distributes glucose to cells for energy and to muscles and liver to be used to form glycogen. Once cells and liver have enough glucose and can't absorb more of it, insulin takes advantage of its connections and acquaintances among enzymes and starts building up fat deposits. The latter happens because we have eaten too much.

In an opposite situation, when we haven't eaten in a while and the glucose levels are low, the pancreas produces glucagon, a hormone with the opposite function to that of insulin. It signals the body to start breaking down the glycogen in muscles and liver into glucose and also triggers a breakdown of fat cells. Attaboy!

The problem is that both of these hormones tend to cancel each other out: when insulin is busy working (the process is called glycolysis), there is no room for glucagon and vice versa. When we're in dietary ketosis, *the opposite* happens.

Because one of the tasks of insulin is storing energy in form of fat supplies and at the same time making sure these fats don't get used, it affects the metabolism of both consumed fats and body fat and it is therefore better if we make sure it isn't busy. Basically it is best kept in the corner, left alone and as quiet as possible. Shoo, you, patron saint of holy fat deposits!

Insulin is, as we've mentioned before, often times confused, but it would be wrong to assume that it is either good or bad: it's confused because of what we put in ourselves. It acts in a way that is best for us in a given moment – the problem is if we, the users of our bodies, make lousy dietary choices. By doing so, insulin can become our long-term nemesis. Take this to your heart and pancreas: do not argue with insulin and don't be teasing it – at least don't do it often.

Numerous types of disease are related to insulin: if we disregard type 1 diabetes, where the body destroys the insulin producing cells in pancreas in an autoimmune reaction that we still haven't found the cause of, along with gestational diabetes, most problems related to insulin are associated with modifiable lifestyle factors and can be prevented.

With an inappropriate diet and a poor lifestyle we put our insulin resistance at risk, a seemingly unnoticeable defect in the regulation of blood sugar levels, which the body is attempting to fix. With time it finds this increasingly harder to do, therefore potentially allowing insulin resistance to develop into type 2 diabetes, metabolic syndrome and all other related issues (none of which are fun to deal with).

Insulin Resistance

As we've already seen, insulin acts as some sort of a janitor, or a local village mailman: when a package arrives, it distributes it throughout the village and villagers are accustomed to open the doors to accept the package and use the content.

However, in certain conditions the villagers refuse to open the door and accept the packages, which then begin piling up clogging the hallways and streets. Pancreas begins producing more insulin, to try and keep on top of things, but the more of insulin there is, the more hesitant and less willing to cooperate villagers become.

In the final phase even pancreas can't produce enough insulin. The blood already contains that much glucose that the condition is identified either as prediabetes or full-blown type 2 diabetes. In the liver, excess glucose is transformed into fatty acids and returned into bloodstream, raising plasma levels of triglycerides and resulting in an increase of fat deposits and a greater risk for development of diabetes and cardiovascular disease.

Insulin resistance, or the resistance of body cells to insulin, is not something we are destined to have, but an acquired disorder. It happens very rarely that the individual is even aware of their insulin resistance, until they are diagnosed with type 2 diabetes because of other present problems. Almost all of the risk factors can be affected with our own decisions. We're putting ourselves at risk if we:

- are overweight;
- have a waist circumference that is too big (31.5 inches for women and 37 inches for men);
- aren't active enough;
- have high blood pressure;
- have low levels of HDL cholesterol
- or if we regularly smoke.

Additional risk factors are cardiovascular disease, family history of diabetes and polycystic ovary syndrome.

Type 2 Diabetes

Type 2 diabetes and its precondition, the insulin resistance, are hard to diagnose since they are slowly and gradually developing conditions. The diagnosis is usually made only once the distinct diabetic complications appear in form of worsened eyesight, hearing, kidney, skin, neurological and cardiovascular issues.

A timely diagnose of a type 2 diabetes can help prevent or delay the onset of complications and is also important as it will enable you to do anything to help your pancreas keep the ability to produce insulin. Long term diabetes can lead to complete inability to produce insulin.

The Metabolic Syndrome

The metabolic syndrome was first mentioned almost 100 years ago, but has only been medically recognized for around a decade. Metabolic syndrome is the name for a number of disorders, all caused by inappropriate and excessive nutrition, lack of physical activity, smoking and similar habits.

In order for this diagnose to be made, the patient needs to have:

• abdominal obesity, determined by waist circumference (31.5 inches for women and 37 inches for men - the risk is considered very big if those numbers are 35 and 40 inches respectively)

and at least two of the following symptoms:
• increased blood levels of triglycerides,
• lowered blood levels of HDL cholesterol,
• high blood pressure,
• increased blood levels of glucose or be already diagnosed with type 2 diabetes.

We often hear of the risk factors from the second section, but we hardly know how serious abdominal obesity actually can be. Although abdominal obesity is more likely to develop in overweight and obese people, it also develops in what seems like individuals with a normal body build.

Abdominal obesity presents a problem because it's not just subcutaneous fat, but fat inside the abdominal cavity. These fat storages on average present as much as 10 percent of all body fat supply.

The Ketogenic Diet, Insulin, Diabetes

There are medication therapies for each of the mentioned metabolic disorders. Once the insulin resistance has been established, the doctor can prescribe medication that will help cells in your body become more susceptible to insulin. Nevertheless, the best treatment and prevention, is a change of lifestyle, mainly a change of diet in order to help insulin do the job it's required to do. Compared to a grandma cruising down the wrong way on a motorway, we simply confiscate its license and car keys.

As we shall later see and as studies also show, we can do this by using a diet with a low carbohydrate and an increased fat intake, or a ketogenic diet – it will be sufficient in some cases, while it will act as a complementary method in others, or as one of the success factors in an integral approach towards fighting disease.

It's worth mentioning that there are no magic methods. For many people, even changing their dietary habits won't be enough. If you were already diagnosed, follow your doctor's instructions and do not reject medication treatment.

Let's do a similar exercise as the one earlier with obesity and ketogenic diet, but this time with insulin and ketones. If we do a search in the Pubmed database for *ketone* and *insulin* or *ketogenic* and *insulin*, we are presented with a continuously growing huge piles of material, from researching the effects of the ketogenic diet on regulating levels of insulin.

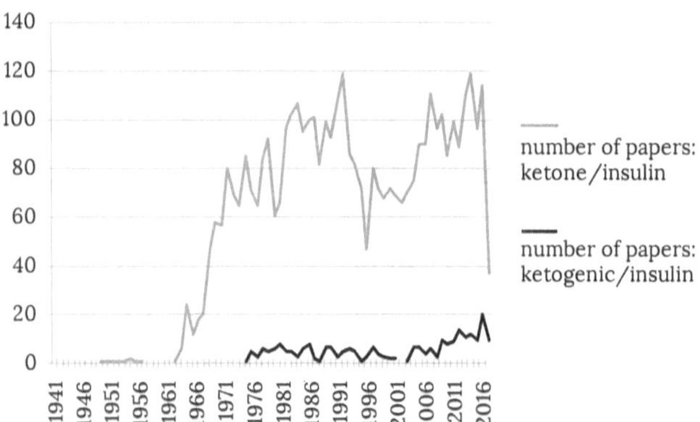

The graph perfectly shows how the words "ketone" and "insulin" appear in scientific documentation in two distinct waves: in the first wave from the mid 60s to the early 90s (the Dr. Atkins diet published in the early 70s is certainly one of the reasons for it) and then again in the new wave, at the beginning of the 21st century. We can't conclude if and how the ketogenic diet or the ketone bodies affect the insulin based just on the number of published documents, but we can see an interest of the scientific community in this subject.

In 2015, a study was published that involved 22 patients with type 1 diabetes, who were prescribed a diet with 70 to 90 grams of carbohydrates daily, while the rest of their energy intake was obtained with fats and protein. The parameters were examined after three and twelve months: there was a significant decrease in occurrence of hypoglycemia per week, the requirement to add insulin after meals was halved, the triglyceride levels were lowered, whereas cholesterol levels remained the same [21].

The effects of the ketogenic diet on the development of type 1 diabetes were also researched in a Swedish study and a recap of this study was published in the *Diabetology & Metabolic Syndrome Magazine*, in May of 2012. 48 patients who couldn't be monitored with any known glycemic methods, were put in a four year educational program on nutrition and diabetes and were at the same time prescribed a diet with a low carbohydrate and a high fat intake. They weren't just trying to see how the diet affects the development of disease, but also whether the patients can stick to it in the long term. They measured the glycated hemoglobin (HbA1C), blood parameter usually above 7 percent in patients with diabetes, at the beginning of the study, four months later and after four years. After two years, approximately half of the participants abandoned the program and the rest successfully followed the program for the full four years. The table below shows results of the measurements of glycated hemoglobin for both groups [22].

	at the start	after 3 months	after 4 years
abandoned after 2 years	7.5%	6.5%	7.4%
4 year program	7.7%	6.4%	6.4%

They specifically focused on a group of 13 individuals who initially had the highest HbA1C (7.8%) and who were the most determined throughout the program: their average final HbA1C value was 6.0 percent! Participants also experienced an improvement in the coefficient between the total and the HDL cholesterol, a known risk factor for development of a heart attack, lowering that risk by 20 percent. Furthermore, the lower HbA1C decreased the risk of cardiovascular disease by 40 percent.

In a study published in 2005 they measured the HbA1C plasma values, triglycerides and cholesterol of 10 overweight patients with type 2 diabetes, after a week of ordinary diet and then again after two weeks of the ketogenic diet. All of the parameters were statistically improved, moreover their insulin resistance after two weeks of ketogenic diet improved by roughly 75 percent!

Even when comparing groups of obese people prescribed with various dietary regimens, similar conclusions were made. Participants achieved good results with as little as 50 percent of their energy intake coming from unsaturated fats – and their insulin levels when fasted dropped to 19 percent. In a group that consumed merely 4 percent of the daily energy intake through carbohydrates and 61 percent through fats (20 percent of which were saturated) the insulin levels when fasted dropped to 33 percent. This group also experienced the biggest drop of triglyceride levels in blood [23].

Studying the effects of the ketogenic diet on overweight people brought similar results. Comparing the two groups of people, where for a period of twelve weeks, one group was using a low carbohydrate intake in combination with 60 percent fat and approximately 30 percent protein, whereas the other consumed a diet of carbohydrates, fats and protein in the 2:1:1 proportion, showed better results in the first group: better body composition, levels of triglycerides and the LDL cholesterol, fasting insulin levels in the first group dropped by almost 50 percent. Furthermore, the researchers noticed a far more substantial loss of abdominal fat in the first group: participants lost on average 828 grams, whereas in the second group this average was 506 grams [24].

Far better metabolic parameters of the group using the ketogenic diet were also discovered in a 2012 study that included 6 months of comparing 58 obese children. One group was prescribed normal nutrition with a restricted energy intake and the other a diet with a drastically lowered carbohydrate intake [25].

There are more and more studies like this. It's worth hoping that experimental and not just observational studies will show what's so far been offering as a possible hypothesis: the ketogenic diet and its effect of lowering and stabilizing blood levels of glucose, can help achieve efficient insulin control, improved insulin resistance and can optimize numerous other parameters known as risk factors for development of too many types of disease, not just diabetes.

Normal levels of key blood parameters in common diet, ketogenic diet and diabetic ketoacidosis are show in the following table.

	common diet	ketogenic diet or dietary ketosis	diabetic ketoacidosis
glucose (mg/dl)	80–120	65-80	> 300
insulin (μU/l)	6-23	6.6-9.4	≅ 0
ketone b. (mmol/l)	0.1	0.3-12	> 25
pH	7.4	7.4	< 7.3

Another review analysis of the current literature should be mentioned, published in the Nutrition magazine in 2014 by a consortium of 26 doctors and dietary researchers (among them were familiar names from the *keto* scene, such as Dr. Richard Feinman, Dr. Eric Westman, Dr. Jeff Volek and Dr. Hussain Dashti). In the analysis they present the fact that despite the tremendous efforts of dietary policies and medicine, diabetes continues to be common and an important pathology. Furthermore, they conclude that the predominant low fat diets are evidently unsuccessful at lowering the obesity epidemic and risks for the development of cardiovascular disease. At the same time they mention the growing material that indicates how diabetes and metabolic syndrome can effectively be regulated with a low carbohydrate diet – without any special side effects. Not just that: they claim that the assumptions on side effects of the low carbohydrate diets are only hypothetical and not factual conclusions based on empirical data. They collectively appeal to the scientific and medical community to reevaluate the current dietary guidelines, using 12 points in which they prove that the low carbohydrate diet should be the first therapeutic approach for type 2 diabetes and an adjuvant therapy to medicinal approach with type 1 diabetes. The review study they claim that:

- carbohydrate restriction is the most effective way of decreasing blood glucose levels;
- the caloric increases, characteristic of the obesity and type 2 diabetes epidemic period, are almost entirely down to an increase in the carbohydrate intake;
- that beneficial effects of carbohydrate restriction occur even without any weight loss;
- even though weight loss is not essential in order to experience beneficial effects of a diet with carbohydrate restriction, the ketogenic diet is still the best of the dietary interventions for weight loss;
- the patients' compliance with type 2 diabetes to the low-carbohydrate diets was at least as good as to any other diets and oftentimes even better;
- swapping carbohydrates with protein is generally beneficial;
- there is no correlation between total dietary and saturated fat and the risk for cardiovascular disease;
- plasma saturated fatty acid levels depend on the intake of dietary carbohydrate much more than they depend on the intake of dietary fat;
- the best predictor of type 2 diabetes complications is glycemic control (HbA1C/glycated hemoglobin A1c);
- aside from starvation, carbohydrate restriction is the best known method for reducing levels of serum triglycerides and raising HDL cholesterol;
- patients with type 2 diabetes who begin using a carbohydrate-restricted diet can often reduce or even eliminate their medication and patients with type 1 diabetes can often lower their insulin doses;
- drastic lowering of the glucose levels by carbohydrate restriction practically has no side effects compared to the intensive pharmacological treatment [26].

Dietary Fats Block Arteries and Are Extremely and Awfully Terrible

No matter who you ask these days, you'll be told that fats are harmful to health (remember Dr. Ancel Keys from the chapter *Obesity Epidemic and Measures to Control it*).

Keys' persecution of dietary fats and his belief that they cause obesity, block arteries and consequently lead to cardiovascular disease was engraved deep in the roots of social consciousness. His theses were supposedly proven by numerous studies in the decades after the condemnation of fat. It would be too strenuous to go into reasons behind society's acceptance of fat as the culprit responsible for all kinds of trouble. It's also hard not to notice that all these years of chasing fats off of menus haven't brought the desired effects, but quite the opposite. Of course, the obesity epidemic isn't solely a consequence of eliminating fats from the menu, but more like a mix of structural and socio-economic circumstances that make us eat more, often cheap food and even more often food with nutritional value unsuitable for the lifestyle that involves less and less physical activity and increasing amounts of stress.

How do we even figure out the effects of food on health and on the development of disease?

In the field of epidemiology the so-called observational studies are used. Most commonly, an observational study consists of large segments of population and establishes patterns between certain environmental factors and their effects on people's health. Epidemiology, like all science, is constantly evolving: research planning, methods, error elimination and determination of correct subject patterns are being improved, thus ensuring increasingly more reliable results. One of the youngest branches of epidemiology is nutritional epidemiology. It has already provided a bunch of solid answers to questions regarding the effects of dietary habits on general health, as well as on particular disease.

This type of research however, has plenty of weaknesses since it is hard to keep in line with controlled clinical studies. When researching the effects of dietary habits, studies usually take time, participants are rarely in a laboratory and isolated from external factors which can disturb the observation processes. It is of course impossible to put people in a laboratory for 10, 15 years and feed them with a concept of a diet that may cause cardiovascular disease. Even if we could put people in a laboratory, this wouldn't be helpful, since we're interested in the results of people living outside of a laboratory, who sometimes fail to eat according to their predetermined dietary concept.

For this reason the nutritional epidemiology uses more or less fitting research methods and statistical models, which help acquire certain results in less time, with less strain for the participants and for less research bucks. Or, as Joanna Blythman recently wrote in the Guardian newspaper, regarding the supposed dangers of red meat consumption: "The dodgy dossier against red meat is based on the shakiest type of evidence: observational studies in which researchers look for patterns in data drawn from notoriously unreliable diet questionnaires." [27]

Even the interpretations of observational studies can be hard to do. There's a more peculiar problem in nutritional epidemiology: statistical models of proportion of food and disease are often focused on individual types of food or macronutrients, but we know that individuals rarely eat just one type of food, or just ONE macro nutrient. These types of studies also rely on personal recollection of participants: the participants in these types of studies use their memory to describe what they consumed and in what amount. You can imagine the nature of errors that appear using this type of data collection.

Another understandable dilemma when it comes to studying effects of a diet on health, is confounding variables: people, who eat healthy are more likely to take better care of themselves in other aspects as well (they are active, they rest more, enjoy things they do ...) In this case, establishing that healthy food is a health factor, isn't entirely accurate. Maybe a mix of beneficial factors and a less reserved approach to living in general, have far more effects on ensuring good health. It is a well known fallacy of the epidemiology studies. Assuming that correlation implies causation is the "false cause", known in Latin *as cum hoc ergo propter hoc* (with this, therefore because of this).

When studying the effects of dietary fats on health and on the risk for developing cardiovascular disease, obesity, diabetes, metabolic syndrome, stroke and similar modern lifestyle "perks" there may have been plenty of these sort of errors. It was during the production of this book that a meta-analysis was published on the effects of butter consumption on the development of cardiovascular disease. All of the analyzed studies involved more than 630,000 individuals and the analysts didn't find any statistically significant evidence of butter consumption affecting the development of cardiovascular disease. In the last five years there has been an increase in meta-analysis rejecting the findings of correlation between consuming saturated fatty acids and developing cardiovascular disease [28].

Or, as the British diabetologist Pamela Dyson opens one of her recent papers: "Dietary treatment of Type 2 diabetes has long been open to controversy and debate, and this is especially true of the relationship between saturated fat and cardiovascular disease. Over the past couple of years, various studies have resulted in headlines claiming that experts have got it wrong for the past 30 years, that there is no link between saturated fat and heart disease, and that healthy diets should include plenty of butter and bacon. ... This has led to much confusion among both people with diabetes and health professionals alike ..." [29].

A controversial question regarding the actual role of fatty acids in the development of cardiovascular disease caused quite a stir among the public and professionals, enough to even get its own Wikipedia page *Saturated fat and cardiovascular disease controversy* (the word controversy was removed on July 24th 2017, though).

Although the debate is ongoing, it's good to know that the knowledge about nutrition is increasing and with it also the means of research, bringing in more reliable results and better knowledge. On top of already mentioned trouble with researching, troublesome interpretation of acquired data, serious and valid division among scientists it is necessary to add that common people have more trouble with science because of uneducated messengers (yes, we're talking about you, newspaper article fillers and creators of hysterical TV content). The media and nutritionists copying each other while seeking sensations and often being intentionally ignorant, incorrectly distribute information and more importantly fail to explain that ONE study does not create DEFINITIVE truth and that the observational study holds far less value than results obtained through controlled experimental studies.

For this reason we emphasize: science is based on the principle of constant examination, repeated research and experiments and most of all the consensus is only reached upon years and years of acquiring irrefutable proof. Smoking is harmful and so are trans-fatty acids.

Extremely and Awfully Terrible Fat
We can confirm one thing: trans-acids are harmful and should be avoided even if you choose a fat rich diet. This conclusion is undisputed and was obtained through aforementioned studies, along with the study about the harmful effects of smoking.

★ *Trans-acids form when any kind of oil is heated, but that's not entirely true: trans-acids form when oil is being overheated and burned. For individuals concerned about their health, one simple rule should be applied. When cooking with fats, make sure not to overheat them and not to overheat them for too long. This is enough to stop us from worrying.*

Most of the trans-acids are in margarine and similar products, as well as products in which margarine is used as an ingredient. Margarine is produced out of vegetable oils, through a process called hydrogenation that changes the position of hydrogen in the fatty-acids molecule. This type of modified fat remains solid or half solid at room temperature and at the same time has longer shelf life.

★ *When food shopping we should always check for hydrogenated or partially hydrogenated fat. We should be careful not just with margarine, but other products as well: many trans-acids are hidden in convenience food, mainly because they are cheap and as such offer a higher profit margin. Read the label on the product packaging and demand information from staff, if you eat out in restaurants and diners. French fries and other deep fried dishes along with mass produced pastry (donuts, croissants, cookies ...) are a rich source of trans-acids.*

Margarine was invented in France at the end of the 19th century, as a substitute for butter and pork fat and became popular during the Second World War due to severe food crisis and high prices of butter.

The human body doesn't need trans-acids. Not only that: consumption of trans-acids disturbs the enzyme function and cuts off the beneficial effects of the good fat we consumed. The general recommendation is: avoid trans-acids like a little puppy avoiding a grumpy old cat. You can even bark at them, but don't try eating them.

Trans-acids also appear in nature and aren't an "invention" we received with hydrogenated oils. Mainly fats of ruminants (also their milk) contain small amounts of trans-acids. It's believed that these aren't harmful to health neither with their structure nor the amount. Furthermore, there exists a special type of CLA fatty acid (conjugated linoleic acid), which has both the trans- and the cis- configuration on various parts of the molecule. Not only is it not harmful, the studies show it is beneficial to health.

One thing needs to be stressed again: no type of carbohydrates are essential for life and health. The body can acquire glucose usually obtained from carbohydrates, through other food sources as well.

On the other hand, some of the fats are essential. This means we *need* to consume them with food. At the same time we can, with quite a high degree of certainly say, that it is more harmful to eliminate fats than carbohydrates from our diet. Unlike glucose, fatty acids play an important role in a number of life processes. As mentioned in the chapters *How does Our Body Get Energy from Food* and *Dietary fats*, fats are a component of cell membranes, nerves and organs; they are the building blocks of hormones, part of the immune system and many other molecules with important body functions; they play an important role in metabolism and providing certain vitamins.

It's also true that distinctively increased values of blood triglycerides and cholesterol aren't good. No one claims they are. The division (see *Dietary Fats Block Arteries and Are Extremely and Awfully Terrible*) among proponents of the ketogenic diet with a high fat intake exists over some of these questions:

• does a high intake of fats cause high values of fat elements in blood or not. Traditionalists claim that the more fat we consume, the more oily our blood will be. Studies show that is it the carbohydrates which are responsible for excess lipids blood, whereas a high intake of fats stabilizes and optimizes the proportion blood lipids;

• are high blood levels of cholesterol a result of an overabundant cholesterol consumption, or an inappropriate diet. You will often hear of the comparison with firemen: where there's a fire, there will soon be firemen. If we go by the traditional definition of cholesterol, then it's obviously the firemen who are starting fires. A more modern definition claims that cholesterol is usually a response to other problems;

• are the reference values for the amounts of HDL and LDL reasonable, or is there any sense at all in constantly lowering these values. "Sense" in this case is health related and it's not about finding sense in pharmaceutical industry maximizing profit by selling statins and other medicine to extinguish the fire, that cholesterol has already come to take care of.

Using Ketogenic Diet to Tame Wild Blood Lipids

One of the most frequently expressed concerns when it comes to a high dietary fat intake diet, is the fear of having increased levels of blood lipids (triglycerides and cholesterol), since these biomarkers indicate an increased risk for a development of cardiovascular disease.

It's a fact that in initial phases of the ketogenic diet, an individual's lipid profile often gets worse at first, but it then later normalizes and improves. If you choose to follow the ketogenic diet it is therefore recommended to regularly monitor your blood count, especially in case you are obese and at risk of developing cardiovascular disease, type 2 diabetes and other similar conditions.

Anecdotal evidence of how some individuals made their blood count immaculate in just a few months, just isn't enough, although it sounds astonishing and has attracted interest of scientific community. The number of studies of the effects a high dietary fat intake has on the blood count is growing daily. This is also clear from the graph showing the number of studies published on PubMed that include these two pairs of keywords "*ketone*" and *triglyceride* and *ketone* and *cholesterol*.

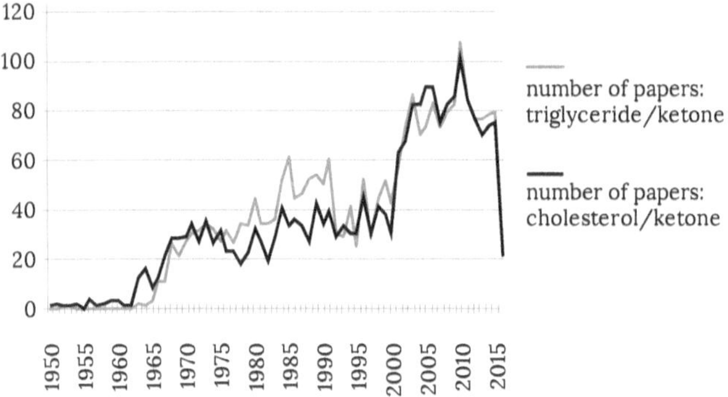

Just as with obesity and insulin, these two word combinations make it obvious that the interest of the scientists in this subject has significantly increased in the last 15 years.

General conclusion of the studies seeking correlation of fat consumption and its effects on lipidogram (a profile of the fat in blood) can be summarized in following statements:

- increased levels of HDL cholesterol;
- lowered levels of triglycerides;
- two different results over total cholesterol in various studies: either no change at all, or an increase in total cholesterol and its stabilization in the upper reference range;
- increased number of large particles of the LDL cholesterol/lowered number of atherogenic, small particles.

In 2002, Eric Westman described the effects of the ketogenic diet on body composition and weight loss, as well as the effects the diet has on the changes of the serum lipid values, in one of the first significant modern studies of ketogenic diet. 51 overweight and obese individuals were prescribed a diet with less than 25 grams of carbohydrates per day and without a prior limitation of the total daily energy intake. Forty-one participants stuck with the diet for the prescribed period of half a year: on average they lost 10 percent of their body weight, roughly 3 percent of it was fat, their levels of total cholesterol, LDL cholesterol and triglycerides decreased, while their HDL cholesterol values increased [31].

Shortly after a study from Kuwait was published, which tried to establish the effects of the ketogenic diet on biochemical parameters. The study involved 83 obese individuals (with a body mass index above 35) with high initial glucose and cholesterol blood values. They were prescribed 24 weeks on a ketogenic diet: 30 grams of carbohydrates, 1 gram of protein per kilogram of body weight, whereas the rest of the energy intake was obtained through 20 percent of saturated and 80 percent polyunsaturated and monounsaturated fatty acids). The results as expected showed a drop of body weight and lower blood levels of total cholesterol, LDL cholesterol, triglycerides and glucose, whereas the levels of HDL cholesterol increased [32].

In 2013, the results of a study carried out in Boston were published in the Metabolism magazine. Two groups of overweight and obese people were monitored for 12 weeks on a low fat and high carbohydrate intake diet (26 individuals) and on a high fat and low carbohydrate intake diet (29 individuals) – both with roughly identical energy intake. Among other things they discovered that the choice of foods affects blood lipids far more than the lowered energy intake. Compared to the low fat intake diet, the high fat intake diet affects blood lipids more favorably: in the group consuming fatty food there was an increase in the levels of HDL cholesterol, a decrease of triglycerides, whereas in the group on a low fat intake diet no changes were registered [33].

To test the belief that eating eggs causes increased blood levels of cholesterol an interesting study was done in 2013. In a randomized, single-blind, parallel design study, a group of 20 individuals consumed 3 whole eggs daily, and in the other group 17 individuals consumed a proportionate amount of egg substitute without the yolk. Both groups consisted of individuals with metabolic syndrome and were on a diet with a moderate intake of carbohydrates (from 25-30 percent of daily energy intake). After 12 weeks results showed that the atherogenic risk due to levels of blood lipids decreased in both groups. Among other things, there was a decrease of blood triglyceride values, small and medium LDL cholesterol particles, an increase in HDL cholesterol and large LDL cholesterol particles, but it was the group consuming eggs that showed better results with HDL cholesterol in particular [34].

In the chapter about the effects of the ketogenic diet on weight loss, we've already mentioned the meta-analysis published in Brazil in 2013, which also showed that the ketogenic diet improves the blood lipid profile and a similar meta-analysis along with a review of existing literature was performed in Canada in 2015. They were looking for a link between consumption of saturated fatty acids and trans-acids and the mortality, occurrence of cardiovascular disease, coronary disease, stroke and type 2 diabetes. An extremely vast review showed that the consumption of fatty acids isn't related to any of the mentioned diseases, although they also established methodological limitations for these claims. On the contrary, they did find a link between the consumption of trans-acids and the mentioned diseases [35].

The Brain Surely Needs Glucose
Proponents of the classic diet pyramid, where the majority of daily energy intake comes from carbohydrates, often claim that the brain cannot function without carbohydrates and that the brain alone requires between 100 to 150 grams of glucose per day. Unfortunately in all those decades of persecuting fats and chasing them off of menus, not many experts were worried about the loss in cognitive and other brain functions because of a distinct deficiency of fats – components of the brain.

To be completely honest, the proponents of carbohydrates are right. When there is an abundance of foods rich in carbohydrates, the brain will happily run on glucose. But as we've seen in the chapter *Fat in the 21st Century: Public Enemy Number 1*, we're currently in a short segment of human history in which any type of food is available in abundance.

So how exactly did humans survive those periods of time when there wasn't enough carbohydrates? Did humans experience a cognitive decline? Of course not. Humans are also fully adapted to foods with low proportion of carbohydrates – even our brain after a certain period of glucose shortage becomes excellent at using ketone bodies. The higher the levels of ketone bodies in our blood are, the more they are being used by the brain. Our brain can get at least two thirds of energy from ketone bodies and the rest from glucose formed through a process of gluconeogenesis (see *How does Our Body Get Energy from Food*).

We could say that humans aren't only fully adapted to foods with a low proportion of carbohydrates. It gets even better: according to the results of studies carried out in the last decade, brain function is even better when using ketone bodies as energy. Although these were individual studies, the findings were interesting:

• dietary ketosis means less oxidative stress for the brain and is therefore protecting the nervous system. Reactive oxygen species accelerate aging processes and are strong risk factors for stroke and nervous system disease and degeneration;

• dietary ketosis improves all kinds of neurological disease by ensuring a more efficient energy supply to brain. This is because beta-hydroxybutyrate, the main ketone bodies (see chapter *Measuring levels of ketone bodies*), provides more energy per unit of oxygen than glucose;

• dietary ketosis promotes biogenesis (formation of new) of mitochondria in hippocampus, a part of the brain crucial for learning and memory;

• if individuals make sure their intake of polyunsaturated fatty acids (mainly omega-3 fatty acids) as part of their ketogenic diet, is sufficient, this beneficially affects the brain, since these fatty acids are the best kind of prevention of inflammatory processes;

• neurons function by excitation and inhibition: the correct proportion between these two modi is regulated by neurotransmitters glutamate (excitatory) and gamma-aminobutyric acid GABA (inhibitory). Too much of glutamate can lead to excitotoxicity and loss of neurons. Excitotoxicity can be a concurrent phenomenon and a factor in stroke, epilepsy and other neurodegenerative disorders. Ketone bodies directly lower the release of glutamate, while increasing the amount of available transmitter GABA – as was shown with some individuals suffering from epilepsy;

• dietary ketosis also affects sleeping: many individuals on the ketogenic diet notice they sleep less, but the quality of their sleep improves. Unfortunately there aren't many decent studies available (especially human studies), however it's been shown in animal models that metabolism of fat, ketone bodies (acetoacetate in particular) and sleep homeostasis are highly related phenomena.

It's worth adding that the ketogenic diet has been a serious subject of scientific discussion for a relatively short period of time and therefore some skepticism is justified.

If we can sprinkle all of that with a pinch of speculation and try to answer the question why dietary ketosis is so beneficial for the brain. Let's look at the pre Neolithic humans, who for the most part didn't grow their food from soil and therefore had to chase animals and catch them in order to get food. Let's say they haven't eaten in a while, their bodies were in dietary ketosis which made them mentally more agile, since their brain was using energy efficient ketones. It seems that this was an evolutionary adaptation that allowed slow two-legged humans to hunt animals more efficiently since animals were faster and more agile. Well, except for sloths, but then again we haven't heard of a sloth stew. It's however true that sloth stew would probably be quite popular today, if western carb loaded men had to catch their food in the wilderness without modern hunting gear and knowledge.

Side Effects

Anything you do could have side effects. It's not clear why they are called side effects, as they are sometimes very direct: you take a sedative and all of a sudden find yourself pleasantly chatting to someone who you normally can't stand.

When reading instruction attached to different medications, the manufacturer informs you of possible side effects: side effects have a certain probability to appear – but aren't compulsory phenomena.

Side effects can also appear when changing dietary habits. In most cases these are temporary effects due to adaptation and they normally disappear after a certain amount of time. While they appear in some cases, many handle the change without any problems – this is a consequence of biological uniqueness (or biological variability) of individuals: although we are very similar, each one of us reacts individually to specific stimuli, with both positive and adverse effects.

Children who spent more time in dietary ketosis because of epilepsy, experienced a side effect in form of bone demineralization, or a decrease in bone density. But it is important to know that children with epilepsy used to be fed with enteral food (liquid concoctions of clinical food) that was evidently lacking minerals. Doctors these days advise children on the ketogenic diet to supplement vitamins and minerals (vitamin D, calcium, magnesium, iron, folic acid) – especially when using liquid concoctions, such as Calogen and Liquigen.

Let's do a comparison: if you go outside in winter, it will be beneficial for you, but there's a chance you will be cold. Will this make you stay inside, or will you simply get dressed more and go outside?

The quality of food we consume is important in every type of diet. Even if you haven't got a specific dietary regimen, it is extremely important to, when possible, choose food of the highest quality. Things aren't any different with the ketogenic diet. If we don't look for shortcuts when choosing foods, we provide our body with everything it needs and more importantly, we avoid potential shortages of micronutrients and consequent health damage those could cause.

If you're hesitant about a high fat diet being right for you, it's good to know that you'll almost definitely experience certain side effects as a consequence of the changes in your diet, which appear in vast majority of individuals who choose the ketogenic diet. Most of them aren't harmful but are simply unpleasant. Fortunately strategies exist that help diminish these effects and help survive the transition to "keto" without any major difficulties. If you're very unsure, consult with your doctor. Only doctors are qualified to give verdicts on whether a chance of a side effect outweighs the chance of a therapeutic effect of a method or medicine.

Keto Flu

The first and most likely problem you may encounter is the so-called keto flu, or a sugar hangover. The chance of you suffering from this sugar hangover a few days upon changing your diet is greater if you consume a lot of carbohydrates, particularly sugar. Withdrawal syndrome could mean headaches, general sickness, fatigue, irritability, low blood pressure – you will feel like you're coming down with flu. An appropriate amount of salt and adding minerals often helps.

Hypoglycemic Episodes

Hypoglycemia is a condition of extremely low levels of glucose in blood, and can feel quite uncomfortable as body releases adrenaline to warn us we must urgently consume food. In involves weakness, tremors or shakes, arrhythmia, vertigo, headache, severe sweating, in extreme cases vomiting, panic attacks and similar symptoms.

When initiating a diet with a low carbohydrate intake, these hypoglycemic episodes are a frequent phenomenon, but it still pays to use certain measures to prevent them from being too frequent and decrease their severity.

There's a higher chance of severe hypoglycemia episodes in people who may be in a prediabetic condition, or who have already developed insulin resistance. Since these two conditions often aren't diagnosed and individuals are unaware of suffering from them, it's good to think about things in detail and plan them out ahead before starting with the ketogenic diet. First of all we have to consider our own existing habits: if we eat a lot of carbohydrates, especially sugar, hypoglycemia is more likely to occur. If the ketogenic diet is drastically different from what you've been eating so far, you should try gradually decreasing the amount of carbohydrates (over a few weeks), before starting with the standard ketogenic diet. If you're unsure on where to begin, consult with an expert in nutrition with a low carbohydrate intake.

For the rest of you the transition will be smoother. If carbohydrates didn't present a large part of your diet, you only have to worry about your meals being frequent enough when starting the ketogenic diet – eat every few hours. Later when you'll already be adapted to using ketone bodies as fuel, these breaks between meals will get longer on their own.

Vitamin and Mineral Deficiency

There's a possibility that by eating food that consists of distinctively small amounts of carbohydrates, you will also consume an insufficient amount of vitamins and minerals, including B-vitamins, magnesium, potassium and sodium. Not necessarily, but it could happen.

Deficiency can be made worse by frequent urination and diarrhea. Furthermore, the lack of vitamins and minerals can be caused by any energy restrictive diet, regardless of what nutrients, proportions and potential cycles the diet prescribes. When choosing foods, it is therefore important to consider diversity and quality.

Shortage of these minerals can be experienced with symptoms similar to those of the keto flu: nausea, unexplained fatigue, anxiety, muscle spasms and shivers, headaches and even arrhythmia. You should plan your diet out so it includes enough eggs, quality butter, broccoli, avocado, salmon, mackerel, anchovy, nuts, natural spices. Don't forget about salt. Yes, you read that right – add salt!

With ketogenic diet you should also make sure that your intake of vitamins A, thiamine (B1), folic acid (B9), C and E, iron and zinc is sufficient.

Frequent Urination

Frequent urination in the first few days of using the ketogenic diet is totally normal and expected. Because of the small intake of carbohydrates, your body begins using glycogen reserves and in doing so, large amount of water is eliminated. More water also gets eliminated because of lower insulin levels: insulin regulates the amount of sodium in a body. Don't forget about the sufficient intake of minerals.

Constipation or Diarrhea

Many fans of the ketogenic diet report of constipation. This usually occurs in the initial phase, namely after dietary changes have been made. Just like with keto flu: the more you change your dietary habits, the higher the chance of experiencing certain adjustment problems will be.

If you were already restricting the amount of carbohydrates before starting the ketogenic diet, you'll probably avoid constipation. Constipation is most likely a result of changes in a diet and will fade out once you adapt to the new diet. It is however more than likely that the amount of stool will be smaller: you will defecate less frequently, in smaller amounts, since you will consume less food that isn't useful to the body.

If you begin to suffer from constipation you need to apply certain measures: have more salt, drink more, occasionally increase your intake of vegetables, especially the kind with seeds, such as cucumber and tomatoes. Adding seeds, such as pumpkin seeds, sesame, chia, and flaxseed, offers relief. Some improve their digestion with running; we don't have to exaggerate, it's enough to simply add a few short but fast sprints to your hike. Adding the MCT oil or coconut butter can also work as somewhat of a laxative.

It's believed that constipation happens because we aren't consuming certain things. But have in mind that constipation can also occur because we eat foods that cause constipation. Try to identify foods which are potentially causing problems, especially if constipation lasts long. Defecation is crucial for health, if you suffer from constipation for longer periods of time you should give serious attention to the issue. Maybe the ketogenic diet isn't for you, or you need special planning of your ketogenic nutrition.

Unlike those with constipation, some can experience diarrhea. This as well can without any doubt be attributed to the change in nutrition. This usually goes away after a few days. It may be that you consume too much protein and not enough fat. When suffering from diarrhea, make sure you stay hydrated and pay special attention to the sufficient intake of minerals (potassium, magnesium and sodium).

If suffering from digestion problems you should also try using shells of psyllium seeds (also known as psyllium husks).

Acetone Breath

Acetone breath is the first sign of uncontrolled diabetes and indicates that the patient may be transitioning into diabetic ketoacidosis and should therefore be treated very seriously. However, with individuals who have just started using the ketogenic diet, acetone breath is common. Once the body runs out of glucose to use as energy, ketone bodies begin forming. As seen in the chapter *Measuring levels of ketone bodies*, we measure one type of ketone bodies, namely acetone, in the exhaled air. Acetone breath is a good indicator that you're in dietary ketosis and going in the right direction. Because the body is adapting to the use of ketone bodies as energy, even bad or fruity breath will disappear – you just have to avoid going on dates during this period. Bad breath can also indicate insufficient levels of sodium, magnesium and potassium, so it's important to ensure that your intake of these minerals is sufficient.

Long-Term Side Effects

There haven't been enough studies of the long-term side effects of the ketogenic diet so we could discuss potential consequences of long-term nutrition based on the ketogenic principles. Despite the accumulation of knowledge regarding the ketogenic diet in recent years, it's hard to speak of a conclusive evidence that the ketogenic diet is safe. There are clinical studies in adults that show that the ketogenic diet is perfectly safe even long term, but as science goes, it's early days yet.

Having said that, however, there is a human population that is more-or-less practicing variations of the ketogenic diet: the inhabitants of the polar regions – the Eskimos, or the Inuit.

A theory exists about a North American Indian tribe Cree, who are Eskimos' Southern neighbors, giving them the name (which they do not like). It apparently derives from the word *askamiciw* ("he eats raw"), in some texts in the language of the Cree tribe, the Inuit are also addressed as *askipiw* ("eats something raw"). Regardless of whether that's true or not, a fact remains that the inhabitants of the Northern regions have traditionally been using the food which was available to them. This was mostly seals, walrus, whales, freshwater and sea fish, Northern terrestrial animals such as caribou, polar bears and musk ox, along with a large amount of cereal.

We're joking. The Inuit barely ever consumed vegetables, especially cereals. If they were lucky enough to find roots or berries, they gladly ate them, but they mostly lived off meat from the mentioned animals, the majority of which have a lot of fat tissue to protect them from the cold environment. Northern hunters didn't just cut that fat tissue away with a pocket knife because they thought fats were horrible, instead, they happily indulged in it. From liver to bone marrow and everything in between. If you have to catch your own food, you simply don't waste any energy rich parts of your catch. Although traditional Inuit diet isn't a homogeneous phenomenon, as it was dependent on the area where Inuit lived, which ranged from Arctic to Subarctic regions of Canada, Alaska, Greenland and Siberia, mostly above the Arctic tree line, it practically didn't involve carbohydrates and rarely involved non-fat meat.

In the 20th century various groups of traditional communities were given quite a lot of scientific attention, but it's clear that most of the knowledge about the effects of traditional diets of Northern people can only be obtained indirectly, since any kind of isolation and authenticity of the Inuit community vanished by mid 20th century. The key was of course the contact with researchers who weren't of Inuit origin: some tribes failed to survive infectious disease, many were modernized. They first abandoned sea food because they established a trade with researchers, then later they abandoned hunting and gathering and started earning wages. Social cooperation, which was required to survive in the wild, was replaced with individualism and traditional foods with supermarket products.

Events based on research and anecdotes, along with plenty of observational studies showed that Inuit traditionally consumed a lot of fish and with that a lot of omega-3 fatty acids. This also explained the small incidence of cardiovascular disease and diabetes in Inuit population. Between 1963 and 1968 the mortality among Greenland's population in cities was higher compared to rural areas, where more traditional dietary habits were preserved. Traditional diet of Northern people relates to high HDL cholesterol levels, low LDL cholesterol levels and low levels of triglycerides. They discovered that consuming seal fat and salmon is linked to a lower risk of impaired glucose tolerance.

In 2000, a group of researchers from Denmark and Greenland published an epidemiological study focusing on diets of 259 adult Inuit, comparing the results to clinical data and blood count of participants. They established a link between sea food consumption and high HDL cholesterol levels and low VLDL and triglyceride levels.

It was by courtesy of the researchers of Arctic cultures that one of most interesting studies of the Inuit diet was created. It was published in the magazine *The Journal of Biological Chemistry*, in 1930. It's not interesting because it included a representative sample of participants, or because it was carried out using modern research methods, but because two westerners – ethnologists and researchers Dr. Vilhjalmur Stefansson and Dr. Karsten Anderson, were fascinated by the Inuit lifestyle (not just by their diet).

After years of living among the Inuit, Dr. Stefansson discovered that he, and his colleagues of European origin, could be healthy and live normally on a typical Inuit diet, consisting of just meat and fish. He was enthusiastic about the Inuit diet and the fact that they never suffered from chronic disease, on top of having extremely beautiful and healthy teeth and was describing his discoveries to scientists in America. They of course just shook their heads full of skepticism. This is the reason behind an interesting experiment in which, Dr. Stefansson, and his colleague Anderson, became test subjects for one year. They consumed only fat rich meat. Dr. Stefansson also occasionally also consumed eggs and butter, if on his lecture trips meat wasn't available. They spent the first few weeks of this diet in a laboratory, afterwards they were living a normal life in New York - while being monitored for the rest of the experiment. After spending a year on the diet, they were examined: blood pressure remained the same in one while the systolic blood pressure slightly decreased in the other, diastolic remained the same as it was before the experiment; neither of them suffered from constipation and they showed no signs of vitamin and mineral deficiency. The tests showed no problems with kidneys. They concluded that a year-long fatty meat diet caused no adverse effects in these two individuals [36].

Until we're certain that long-term use of the ketogenic diet is a good thing, we can either take the risk, or use an intermediate approach. A group of Italian scientists, led by the professor Antonio Paoli for instance suggests we should perform cycles of ketogenic and Mediterranean diet, where the ketogenic diet cycle is shorter and the Mediterranean diet cycle can last up to a few months. It's a fact that at professional conferences dedicated to ketogenic diet, speakers are always slim, healthy, youthful looking people full of vitality, despite being over 50 or even older.

Who is the Diet Rich in Fats Suitable for?

With this next statement, the authors risk being accused of living in a bubble. No one tells you anything, but then while chitchatting about this and that it turns out that a bunch of people around you silently suck on cubes of butter and sip on buckets of double cream for breakfast. We almost don't know anyone who doesn't do the "fat fad" anymore.

But are diets of ketogenic nature suitable for everyone?

There is no unambiguous answer to that, mostly because there aren't enough definitive scientific conclusions and because some co-effects have not been studied properly yet (for example, the effect of a ketogenic diet on thyroid and thyroid hormones). The most accurate answer we can give to that question is: yes and no.

As long as you're healthy there's no reason you shouldn't try using even the strictest variation of the ketogenic diet for a specific time period. However, even with healthy people we don't yet know for sure if long-term use of ketogenic diet is appropriate and can be considered as a life dietary strategy. This doesn't mean it's inappropriate – but just that we don't yet know if it's appropriate. There are clinical studies that confirm the notion that the ketogenic diet is effective, safe and with only a few side effects, that appear to be of a transient nature. Additionally, a lot of anecdotal evidence exists – but as you already know – that's not science. Science demands years long observations, repetitions and so on. The initial body of evidence, however, looks promising.

In case you're having doubts, or suspect you might suffer from a serious medical condition, you should consider the following options before you start living off pork cracklings on butter, piled on top of avocado and dressed with cocoa coconut balls:

• consult your personal doctor. Since there's a high chance that your personal doctor won't be familiar with the potential of the ketogenic diet, you should try and find a doctor who's informed of the modern nutritional studies;

- inform your doctor of your intention and ask them for assistance in your effort;
- ask if you can have blood tests carried out at the expense of insurance company; if you can't, pay for it yourself and ask the doctor to monitor and interpret your blood count (fasting insulin and glucose, lipid profile, kidney tests, thyroid hormones, if needed also minerals, vitamins and C-reactive protein);
- don't just jump in with the strictest variation of a ketogenic diet (roughly 20 grams of carbohydrates per day), instead begin gradually: lower your carbohydrate intake to around 100 to 150 grams daily, which you will make up for with a higher intake of fats. If everything goes well, keep lowering the amount of carbohydrates and increasing your intake of fat;
- consider using one of the methods for measuring levels of ketone bodies;
- monitor yourself, and pay attention until you're absolutely certain that a higher fat intake isn't harmful for your existing medical problem.

Ketogenic type of diets definitely aren't suitable for people with lipid metabolism disorders and those of you suffering from such disorders, hopefully know that already. Despite the abundance of existing literature regarding beneficial effect of ketogenic diets on the course of type 1 diabetes, caution is advised with these sort of patients – if you suffer from type 1, it is urgent you consult any changes to your diet with a doctor. Same goes for those with kidney problems, gout or those susceptible to gout, and those with cardiovascular disease.

Sometimes these type of diets prove not to go very well even with healthy individuals. Individuals might love carbohydrates the most out of all foods. It's possible that after a certain amount of time on the ketogenic diet, even that relationship would come to an end, but the psychological pressure might be unbearable.

Certain side effects of a fat rich diet affect some people significantly more compared to the majority. Some endurance athletes have to adapt their ketogenic diet to sport. Athletes generally have to be specific at maintaining their muscle mass – when opting for the ketogenic diet, things need to be thought through and designed individually.

Diets based on ketogenic processes have certain effects and are suitable for those who wish to achieve these effects – in principle, anyone. We have introduced three processes in detail, which can be affected beneficially based on the principles of a ketogenic diet: weight loss, insulin regulation and regulation of blood lipid profile. If those three factors are balanced, we have drastically lowered the risk for a development of metabolic syndrome, type 2 diabetes, cardiovascular disease and supposedly a whole other bunch of problems. We have also given some attention to the effects of the ketogenic diet on the functioning of the nervous system, or brain.

As we've mentioned a few times already, the ketogenic diet and its effects are still widely studied and researched, hence it's too soon to declare any undeniable truths (yet). Experience and studies so far describe the following effects of fat rich diets:

• a balanced proportion of all key blood biomarkers (glucose, triglycerides, proportion of LDL and HDL cholesterol, an increase in the amount of large LDL cholesterol particles);

• ketone bodies have an anorexic effect (don't panic, the word anorexic in this case means it reduces the sense of hunger, i.e. lowers appetite);

• balanced glucose levels beneficially affect the proportion between insulin, glucagon and epinephrine, providing good conditions for lowered lipogenesis and increased lipolysis (in layman's words: less fat deposit formation and more energy release from the existing fat deposits);

• a favorable mix of factors for lowering a risk for development of insulin resistance, metabolic syndrome, type 2 diabetes, high blood pressure, cardiovascular disease;

• high levels of ketone bodies and short-chain and medium-chain fatty acids in blood, evidently benefit nervous and hormone systems and increase mental agility of individuals;

• using ketone bodies as energy instead of glucose reduces the level of oxidative stress and inflammatory response which can slow down aging of tissue and potentially the development of cancer[3].

Dilemma: Keto or LCHF?

The difference between the ketogenic and LCHF diet is that with the latter we get to determine the minimum amount of carbohydrates we wish to intake. The carb range is generally up to 100 grams daily. LCHF allows a bit more vegetables, nuts and occasionally even a piece of chocolate and similar foods. LCHF diet also allows us to more loosely determine the proportion of consumed fats and protein, although the focus still remains quite a substantial intake of dietary fats.

---

3   A few genuine indicators show that beta hydroxybutyrate, a ketone body, functions the same way as a group of the latest cancer medications, which act as HDAC inhibitors. It also seems that regulation of insulin release, or dietary ketosis, is an efficient concomitant therapy for cancer patients. Another option for future evolution of medicine within oncology is based on the observation that shows some cancer cells being unable to use ketones as energy and depend on glucose.

Let's say that the difference between the ketogenic diet and LCHF is something like the difference between the Shanghai Maglev magnetic levitation train, which travels 19 miles in 7 minutes, and the Eurostar train, which travels from Brussels to London in an hour and forty five minutes. The first one isn't exactly comfortable, since it doesn't drop passengers of in the center of Shanghai, whereas the other is a bit slower, but more user friendly, since you can board it in the center of Brussels and you can get off in the center of Paris or London.

As it currently seems, all other dietary regimens are somewhere on the level of third world country railways. While they do get you to the location eventually, they make you lose the will to travel on the way there. Unless you're Gašper Grom, who makes use of the time on trains by replying to your questions regarding the ketogenic and LCHF diets.

So? If you've made the decision to give high fat diet a go, you need to ask yourself, how strict of a regimen you are willing to set. The ketogenic diet is stricter, brings faster results, while the LCHF offers more flexibility, less initial issues and at the same time makes changes to your body less rapid and drastic. It seems you need a bit of self-assessment to figure out what you want and how much you're willing to invest to get there.

Regardless of your desires and readiness to try the keto, we recommend a gradual approach, especially if you're used to a high carbohydrate intake. Quick change of a diet can cause an illness, which we fondly call the keto flu.

Keto Ratios – Ratios of Macro Nutrients

The difference between using the LCHF and the ketogenic diet is shown schematically in the table below[4].

foods	carbohydrates	protein	fats
LCHF	25–130 g	20–30% DEI*	70–80% DEI
(standard) ketogenic	less than 20 g and no more than 50 g	10–20% DEI	80-90% DEI

* DEI: daily energy intake

We should mention that the presented ratios are in a way theoretical, since there isn't an ideal and accurate proportion that would work for everyone.

We're all different – some of us need to lower the amount of carbohydrate down to a minimum, again others will be successful with a less strict measuring. The amount of fats and protein also depend on gender, body weight, body composition and also on physical activity. For some extremely active individuals it is possible to increase the prescribed amount of 25 grams and adapt it to fit the sport schedule.

You will sometimes come across the term "keto ratio" or "keto macro". Keto ratio is the ratio between the energy value of fat intake in grams compared to the energy value sum of protein and carbohydrates in grams. Although a 5:1 ratio diet is possible, when describing the standard ketogenic diet we usually speak of a 4:1 ratio – meaning: for every gram from protein and carbohydrates combined,

---

4 We wanted to add the latest recommendations of government organizations for comparison: the well known American diet pyramid, first published in 1994, was in 2011 replaced with the concept of »my plate« (MyPlate), consisting of fruit, cereals, vegetables, protein and dairy products, not giving fats any special place on the plate and when speaking of fats, it recommends keeping their intake at a minimum and choose low fat foods, less fatty meat parts etc.

we add 4 grams of fat. The ratios can also be lower: 3.5:1 or 3:1 and lean more towards the direction of LCHF.

Since keto ratio isn't just a theoretical construct and is determined according to our needs, habits and goals, we will give it more attention when we'll be talking about the actual use of the ketogenic diet.

We have to mention another two types of ketogenic diet.

In our standard introduction of the ketogenic diet, we presented it as a diet with a daily intake of under 20 grams of carbohydrates (or a maximum of 50 grams, depending on the type of individual), however, there are two more approaches, which are based on adding carbohydrates to what is otherwise a ketogenic diet:

• targeted ketogenic diet: this type of diet involves planning a daily meal with an increased intake of carbohydrates around exercise;

• cyclical ketogenic diet: consists of a defined interval day (usually once weekly), when by consuming meals rich in carbohydrates we replenish glycogen reserves. As a side note: Dr. Jeff Volek showed in his research with ultra-marathoners and ironman distance triathletes that patterns of glycogen depletion during exercise and replenishment post exercise had less variability with chronic keto-adapted elite athletes than the same processes with athletes who were on high carb diet [37].

PRACTICAL ADVICE

You're already familiar with the theory behind the ketogenic diet (especially since you've read the first part of the book), now it's time to get things rolling. Practical advice is given in form of questions and answers that will guide your life through the maze of the ketogenic diet. Are you ready?

- **How to know where to start?**

You've already read who the ketogenic diet is suitable for, who needs to be cautious and consult a doctor, you also know that practicing the ketogenic diet will include eating things you previously considered as harmful.

Start by assessing your dietary habits.

How will you survive your first ten days on a ketogenic diet (you start tomorrow, right?) will mostly depend on your current diet – and by current, we mean your current high-carb diet. Of course survival of the adaptation period can be regulated on the go, but how you set things up can also be of importance.

It does sometimes happen that people bail on their ketogenic diet before ever achieving ketosis. The whole power of the ketogenic diet comes to show with a similar delay to that of antidepressants. While it at first may seem like nothing, or you may even feel nauseous and irritable, things then in a period of 10 to 14 days – completely turn around.

How difficult the adaptation period will be for you – as already stated – largely depends on your previous diet. The question here is not whether you're in a constant energy surplus, but what in what proportion your consumed macronutrients are. If you eat ordinary foods, in this case "ordinary" stands for Western diets, where breakfast consists of bread or cereal, lunch of rice or pasta, snacks consist of fruit and chocolate and dinner of rice pudding or grits, then you need to choose a different strategy than someone who follows a fitness menu with a low intake of carbohydrates and fats along with a high intake of protein.

If carbohydrates present an important part of your diet, you have two options; you either gradually prepare for a low intake of carbohydrates by lowering their intake for a week or two, or you simply bite the bullet from the get go and deal with the drastic reduction. Gradation techniques are up to you, but here's a suggestion: in the first week, reduce the carbohydrates to a half of what you usually have and in the second week, go even further and consume only a third of your usual carb intake. Afterwards the transition to a keto carb reduction should be smooth.

Just a heads up: if you switch from a high carb diet to LCHF overnight, you're at far greater risk to experience keto flu (see chapter *Keto Flu*): don't let this scare you or stop you from continuing. Just remember: adding salt and other minerals will diminish the chances of keto flu.

◆ OK, I know what I eat, what now?

First you need to clean your kitchen and pantry. And your drawer with sweets in your office desk. You need to get rid of all carbohydrates.

Begin with basic foods: sugar, flour, all kinds of cereals, pasta, rice, polenta, grits, bread, breadsticks, crackers, all kinds of bread substitutes such as rice cakes, puff pastry, phyllo pastry, pizza dough. Don't forget to chuck away those bread crumbed chicken fillets and the like out of your freezer. Tuberous vegetables such as potatoes, carrots are allowed to stay but not a full year's supply, but just a piece or two. Maybe just one piece. Same goes for legumes.

All sweets must go: candies, cookies, pies, sweet rolls, chocolate, chocolate eggs, pastry, cakes. You also won't be needing any salty snacks such as potato chips, cornmeal snacks and pretzels. Sugary drinks, juice, beer and similar things are out of the question. And that's not everything: in the initial phase you should stay away from anything sweet – even from sweets that contain sugar substitutes and have no calorie value.

Once you successfully achieve dietary ketosis and mentally calm down you can slowly incorporate those things again. You will even be able to indulge in small portions of dark chocolate or sugar free chocolate (it's also likely that you won't even crave chocolate anymore). Furthermore, there are countless options and products on the market today to satisfy the needs of those with a sweet tooth without interrupting ketosis. Caution against saccharin, aspartame and sucralose. These have been shown in an animal study to disrupt the gut microbiome and in doing so, can lead to insulin resistance [38, 39].

Fruit. Eat what you have today or give it to someone because you won't be needing it. You can keep a lemon and a few berries if necessary. The rest of it is out of the picture.

If your fridge is full of low fat products you don't have to discard them, but do stop buying them.

Now that everything is tidy, purchase the following foods in this sort of order: eggs, butter, coconut butter, olive oil, avocado, fish, fatty meat pieces (sausages, bacon, lard, pork cracklings), sour and double cream, fatty cheese, some full fat cottage cheese, a lot of green and leafy vegetables and nuts, such as macadamia, hazelnuts and almonds.

You can of course also buy white and lean meat, but in that case you need to throw in at least 2 more pounds of butter and olive oil. Buy quality salt.

If possible buy locally produced foods of the highest quality, and organic when possible – even when not on ketogenic diet.

◆ **Why do things have to be so strict right at the start? Wouldn't it be easier if we transitioned to a ketogenic menu slowly and gradually?**

This is down to individuals, but since a large majority of people who decide to use the ketogenic diet, experience trouble with controlling their appetite and fighting cravings, it is recommended to begin in this strict manner and give up treats. This isn't that hard to do when using the ketogenic diet, as appetite often drops and most people do not experience the familiar feeling of "dietary" restraint.

Once we get used to the new dietary habits, there's nothing wrong with occasionally indulging in keto sweets (such as those found in the LCHFlove.com's recipe section, you can find the link to it in the final chapter), coffee with double cream or sugar free soda (if you simply have to drink this "health elixir").

♦ I'm meant to eat that white stuff on prosciutto? Are you two a bit crazy?

Butter on eggs, lard on pancetta, pork cracklings on avocado, bacon roll with cheese and so on. This is the ketogenic diet.

There are a lot of us who needed quite a lot of mental preparation to swallow down a piece of bacon roll without experiencing inner drama, or to pick the bacon piece with more "white stuff" instead of the meaty one. Take into account that your plan of transitioning to dietary ketosis will be somewhat hindered by the mentality we've force fed ourselves with for decades.

♦ What amount of carbohydrates should I plan at the beginning?

It can be done cold turkey style, which means lowering carbohydrates to approximately 5 percent of your daily energy intake, or somewhere between 20 to 30 grams per day, but we still recommend you start the first week or two with more, around 10 percent of daily energy intake which means approximately 40 to 70 grams. You will obtain these carbohydrates from nuts and vegetables, mainly leafy types.

Avoid starchy vegetables, or at least consume them in minimal amounts.

You might eventually start noticing that you manage to stay in dietary ketosis even with a higher intake of carbohydrates, while you still get to enjoy all the benefits of a ketogenic diet. This is totally possible and also OK.

If you can stay in ketosis despite a higher intake of carbohydrates, it most probably indicates that you have no problems with insulin resistance of cells.

- **How much protein?**

The ketogenic diet – as mentioned before – isn't a high-protein diet, therefore you shouldn't consume too much protein.

The best rule is to consume as many grams of protein as your bodyweight is in kilograms, or even a bit less than that. If you have 75 kilograms, the right amount of protein will be between 60 and 75 grams. They should account for approximately 20 percent of daily energy intake, which means between 50 and 130 grams, depending on your weight as well as your physical activity. Those who are physically active can use the upper limit of the recommended amount of protein.

- **What about fats?**

The rest of what you consume should be fats. If possible they should be of animal origin (egg yolk, meat, butter). You should also use coconut butter, olives and olive oil, avocado and avocado oil, hazelnuts, macadamia oil and nuts.

- **OK, it seems that you're telling me to count calories and weigh foods. I'm not too keen on that.**

Yes and no. If you were already disciplined with food before and you have a sense of proportion of macronutrients in specific foods, you won't have any problems. If you don't already have a sense of amounts and proportions it would be useful to get familiar with these things. You can use any kind of tool that shows macro- and micro-nutritional composition of particular food – there are a lot of them online in many languages. Most products have their composition listed on the packaging. The time you invest in learning characteristics of food will be paid off in spades: a slim body, health and wellbeing.

When we say that you need 20 grams of carbohydrates daily, this doesn't mean 20 grams of salad, but usually a lot more. There is only one type of food where its weight matches the weight of the carbohydrates it contains and that's sugar. Examples of 20 grams of carbohydrate:

- approximately 600 grams of iceberg lettuce;
- almost 900 grams of Chinese cabbage;
- approximately 90 grams of almonds.

You have to count all of the consumed carbohydrates, not just those in vegetables. Almonds are a good example of foods that are primarily composed of fat but also contain carbohydrates. Pay special attention to condiments – if you use a lot of balsamic vinegar you should for instance be aware that 100 grams of vinegar contains 17 grams of carbohydrates.

But we have some good news: if a type of food contains a total of 20 grams of carbohydrates and 7 grams out of those are fiber, you only add 13 grams towards your daily count. Fiber doesn't need to be counted as consumed carbohydrates.

A similar measuring exercise needs to also be done with protein and fat. The food usually weighs more than the prescribed nutrient. Foods with one predominant nutrient are rare, but they do exist, for instance all oils (100% fat content), whey powder (from 70 to 90% of protein), butter (80% fat)...

- **Can I avoid fat?**

You can, if you can survive on 20 grams of carbohydrates and roughly 100 grams of protein per day. No, of course not! Fats need to be eaten and shouldn't be avoided: they are not optional, but obligatory.

- **Understood. 20 to 30 grams of carbohydrates, 50 to 130 grams of protein, and as much fat as I can stuff myself with?**

Yes and no.

An intake of fat that is too high will be counterproductive. At the beginning your appetite might change, it might even increase, but once your body gets accustomed to a low carbohydrate intake and with that starts to run on energy from fats, the appetite will calm down again. This means that in time, you will be eating the right way without any specific dietary "satellite navigation" and "calculation". Most likely you will be less hungry, won't be craving food as much and will consequently eat less – without putting in effort and or paying attention. It happens that people decrease the number of their meals because they are simply too full.

- **Does it matter if I'm a petite woman or a 265 lbs and 6'6 tall man when determining the amount of carbohydrates and protein?**

Of course it matters. How can we make things easier? By using online questionnaires and calculators we can determine the required daily energy intake and based on it establish our requirements with specific nutrients.

Let's use the typical ratio of a standard ketogenic diet 5% : 20% : 75% (CHO : P : F). A petite woman, who spends most of her time sitting down, will most likely need around 1,500 kcal energy daily.

The table shows that according to the standard ketogenic diet, she will have to consume 19 grams of carbohydrates, 56 grams of protein and 133 grams of fats. Her 6' 6" male colleague, who also regularly plays sports might need between 2,300 and 3,000 kcal which makes the amount of required nutrients a lot higher.

keto ratio	5%	15%	80%
kcal	CHO (g)	P (g)	F (g)
1,500	19	56	133
1,700	21	64	151
2,000	25	75	178
2,300	29	86	204
2,500	31	94	222
3,000	38	113	267

◆ **A proportion of 5% : 20% : 75% (CHO : P : F) the only savior?**

No, just the most typical. There are no fixed numbers of ratios we should consume to stay in dietary ketosis, however, it is estimated that to achieve ketosis a minimum of 60 percent of daily energy intake has to come from fat (along with a small amount from carbohydrates).

The tables below show a few more possible ratios, including their amounts of macronutrients calculated according to the daily target energy intake.

Which one to pick? For people with insulin resistance, or prediabetes, it's recommended to lower the amount of carbohydrates as much as it's possible. Those who live an active lifestyle might choose a model with a slightly higher amount of carbohydrates.

It is also possible to test things yourself: start with the lowest possible intake of carbohydrates and upon achieving ketosis try to raise the amount if this suits you.

If you still manage to achieve your goals, even with more carbohydrates and if this suits you, then there's no reason to stick to the strictest form of ketogenic diet.

keto ratio	5%	15%	80%
kcal	CHO (g)	P (g)	F (g)
1,500	19	75	125
1,700	21	85	142
2,000	25	100	167
2,300	29	115	192
2,500	31	125	208
3,000	38	150	250

keto ratio	10%	15%	75%
kcal	CHO (g)	P (g)	F (g)
1,500	38	56	125
1,700	43	64	142
2,000	50	75	167
2,300	58	86	192
2,500	63	94	208
3,000	75	113	250

keto ratio	10%	20%	70%
kcal	CHO (g)	P (g)	F (g)
1,500	38	75	117
1,700	43	85	132
2,000	50	100	156
2,300	58	115	179
2,500	63	125	194
3,000	75	150	233

- **But I really can't be dealing with all these numbers!** It's totally understandable that there are too many instructions for you to follow them all. Some of you have exhausting jobs and simply seek instructions on what, when and how much to eat. Find a nutrition expert in ketogenic or LCHF diets. Gašper, the co-author and the mastermind behind LCHFlove.com has so far helped over a thousand individuals to lose weight and restore their health.

+ **What should I focus on in the first few weeks?**
Before achieving metabolic transition, you may encounter some transient problems (see chapter *Side Effects*). If you're hungry eat eggs, a spoonful of pork cracklings, and have coffee with butter. Take into account that you're in a period of adaptation. Don't lose hope, even if you exceed your daily target energy intake. Your first objective in the initial weeks is not to give up and not to increase the intake of carbohydrates.

+ **Can I eat porridge / granola?**
You can, half a teaspoon per 3 days. If you intend on using the ketogenic diet, then porridge (pizza, bread, rye meal ...) is out of the question. However, the ketogenic diet isn't mandatory. Some people normally live off porridge and curdled milk and they aren't fat or suffer from disease.

Luckily, there are LCHF/keto porridge recipes that you can make yourself. They typically include a combination of roasted hazelnuts, coconut crisps, hemp seeds, chia seeds, flaxseeds, chopped dark chocolate, cinnamon – with added butter, coconut oil and MCT oil to meet the fat requirement.

+ **Can I get some basic recipes to start things easier?**
One of the advantages of the ketogenic diet is the simplicity of meal recipes. Even if we don't prepare food in advance, this is the simplest way to consume food, as my co-author, who spent years creating fitness meals assures. If we have a fridge available (at work for example), then there really is no problem.

On the other hand the ketogenic diet is also a diet that allows a lot of experimenting in the kitchen and is very practical from that point of view. While there is no pasta, rice, pies and bakers' wares, there are stews, soups, roasts – things that can be prepared in advance, for multiple occasions.

Here are just a few quick ideas since accurate recipes are beyond this book's purpose:

- fried eggs with butter and spinach;
- hardboiled eggs with cheese;
- fried eggs with pork cracklings;
- a piece of full fat cheese with nuts;
- bacon (fried or not) with a spoon of almond butter;
- lard on cheese slices with pickled cucumbers;
- grilled salmon with Swiss chard and butter;
- protein shake mixed in with double cream;
- a spoon of full fat cottage cheese with plenty of sour cream;
- a spoon of full fat cottage cheese with double cream and some almonds;
- lettuce with half of avocado, fried chicken, a bit of tomato and olive oil.

Use spices. These enrich dishes and make them taste delicious and look appealing. You can find plenty of useful recipes in the LCHFlove.com's kitchen at: *http://www.lchflove.com/lchf-recipes/*

- **What does an example of a menu look like?**

Once you're "on board", assembling menus for the ketogenic diet becomes easy. Here are two examples of a menu: Judging by the experience of numerous users, it is best to start with three, rarely with four meals; once in ketosis usually even three meals become too much and most end up consuming two meals daily. Most often people report about not feeing hungry in the morning, so they start skipping breakfast altogether. There is nothing wrong with that: once the body becomes accustomed to using fatty acids and ketone bodies as energy, the lack of hunger in the morning is completely normal.

An example of a three meal menu

breakfast	kcal
4 eggs (large)	286
30 grams of butter	201
150 g of parboiled spinach	35
lunch or a snack	
120 g of Gouda cheese	428
75 g of hazelnuts	472
dinner	
1 avocado (approx. 140 g)	227
150 g of chicken breast	258
1 mid size tomato	22
100 g of broccoli	28
200 g of endive	30
	1,987

An example of a two-meal menu

lunch	kcal
3 eggs (large)	214
30 grams of butter	201
50 g of pork cracklings	286
50 g of Parmesan cheese	201
dinner	
200 g salmon fillet	284
4 spoons of olive oil	476
1 large zucchini, grilled (approx. 300 g)	48
	1,711

◆ **A list of appropriate foods**

Choose foods, marked with ❶ and ❷ on everyday basis. Make sure you add some butter or olive oil to the meat and fish in the category ❷. Foods marked with ❸ and ❹ are OK, but should for different reasons only be eaten occasionally or in very small amounts.

Eggs

❶ eggs

Fatty foods

❶ butter (from cow milk, buffalo milk, goat milk …) or clarified butter (ghee)

❶ hazelnuts, macadamia nuts

❶ avocado

❶ fish oil, coconut oil, avocado oil, hazelnut oil, olive oil

❷ mayonnaise (homemade and on olive oil basis)

Meat

❶ fatty turkey, fatty chicken, fatty pork, fatty lamb, fatty beef / veal

❷ chicken breast – luncheon variant (low fat), rabbit, bear, goat, lean veal, horse, boar, lean turkey, lean pork, hare, lean beef, lean chicken, deer

❸ high quality homemade sausages, pork cracklings

Fish & Seafood

❶ salmon, mackerel, herring, sardines, halibut

❷ tuna (bluefin), yellowtail, hake, shark, trout, anchovy, swordfish, pollock, perch, striped mullet, pike, whitefish species, squid

❸ sea bass, herring, carp, seatrout, squid / calamari

Dairy

❶ hard goat cheese, Gruyère, Emmental, Cheddar, Parmesan, pecorino, fontina, Edam, Gouda, blue cheese
❷ heavy cream (30% fat)
❷ sour cream (20% fat)
❷ Brie, Limburger, Camembert, whole milk mozzarella, feta, goat soft cheese, Neufchatel
❸ whole milk ricotta
❹ cottage cheese, cream cheese, Greek yoghurt

Vegetables

❶ watercress, Chinese cabbage, lettuce, pickles, celery, zucchini, white mushrooms, endive, radishes, spinach, cucumber, arugula, Swiss chard, asparagus, chicory, radicchio, rhubarb, green peppers, chicory greens
❷ tomatoes, capers, cauliflower, green tomatoes, banana pepper, cress, young onion greens, cabbage, eggplant, red peppers, green cauliflower, kohlrabi, yellow peppers, turnips, pumpkin, broccoli, spring onions, red cabbage
❸ snap beans, okra, baby carrots, kale, Brussels sprouts, dandelion greens, celeriac, onions, beets, carrots
❹ squash, leeks, shallots, ginger root, parsnips

Other

❷ olives
❹ casein based protein supplement
❹ almonds, walnuts, pecans, peanuts, brazil nuts …

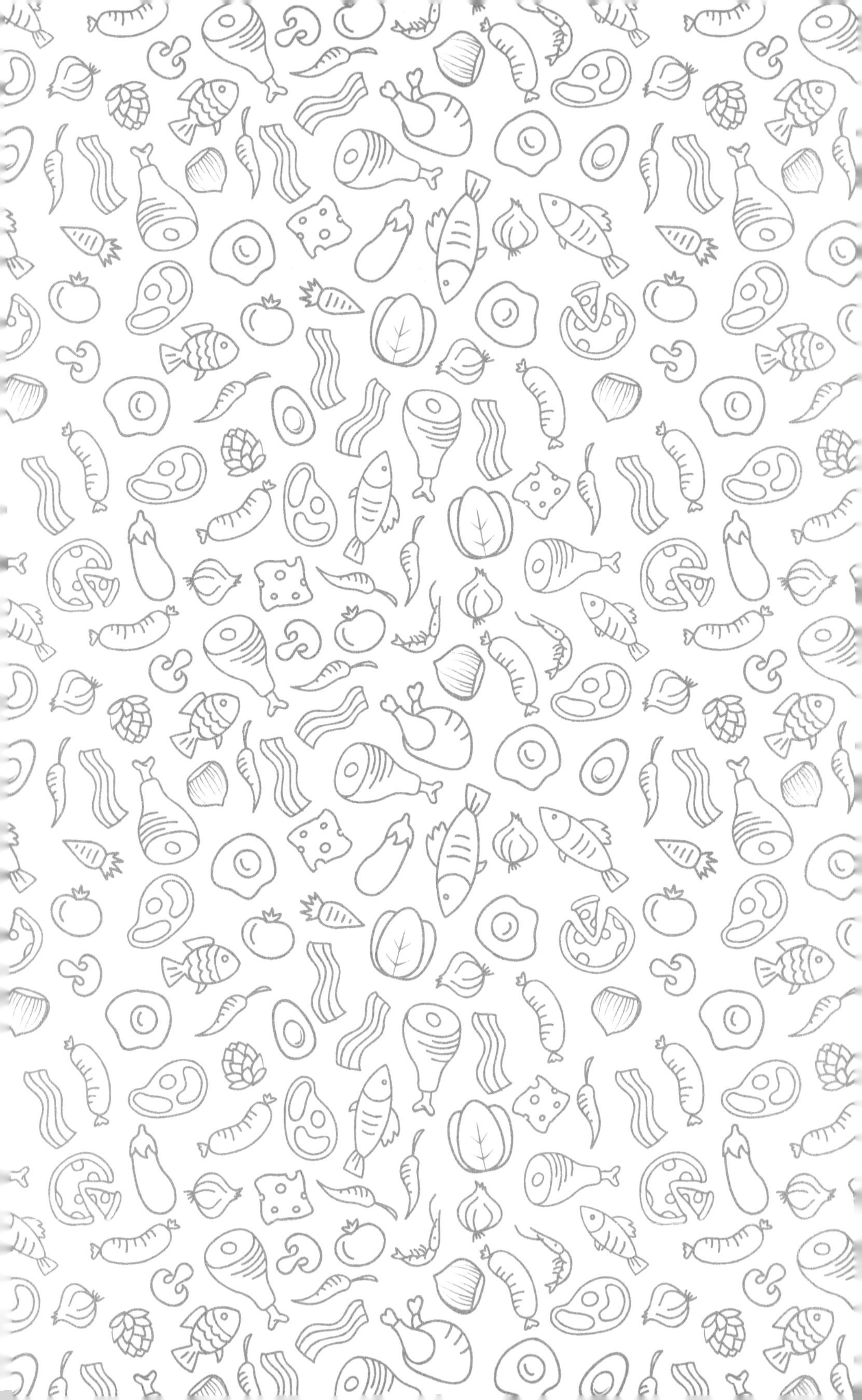

FINAL THOUGHTS

Worrying about eating properly and seeking healthier alternatives only makes sense to the point where it becomes a burden and triggers a state of constant anxiety with everything occurring anywhere between hands – and mouth. Nutrition needs to be loosened, food needs to be enjoyed and we shouldn't allow our heads to be filled with concepts of sin, guilt and self-inadequacy because of food. Whenever we are displeased, whether this derives from our appearance, moral guilt for committing "a sin" by eating something we shouldn't have, we are more susceptible to messages that reinforce these convictions and pull us into a vicious circle of constant stress and its harmful consequences. Many of us who have gone through these phases discovered that fat rich food helps relax the hectic psychological dynamic humans evolved towards food, restores health and makes life more beautiful.

We wish that you also achieve this.

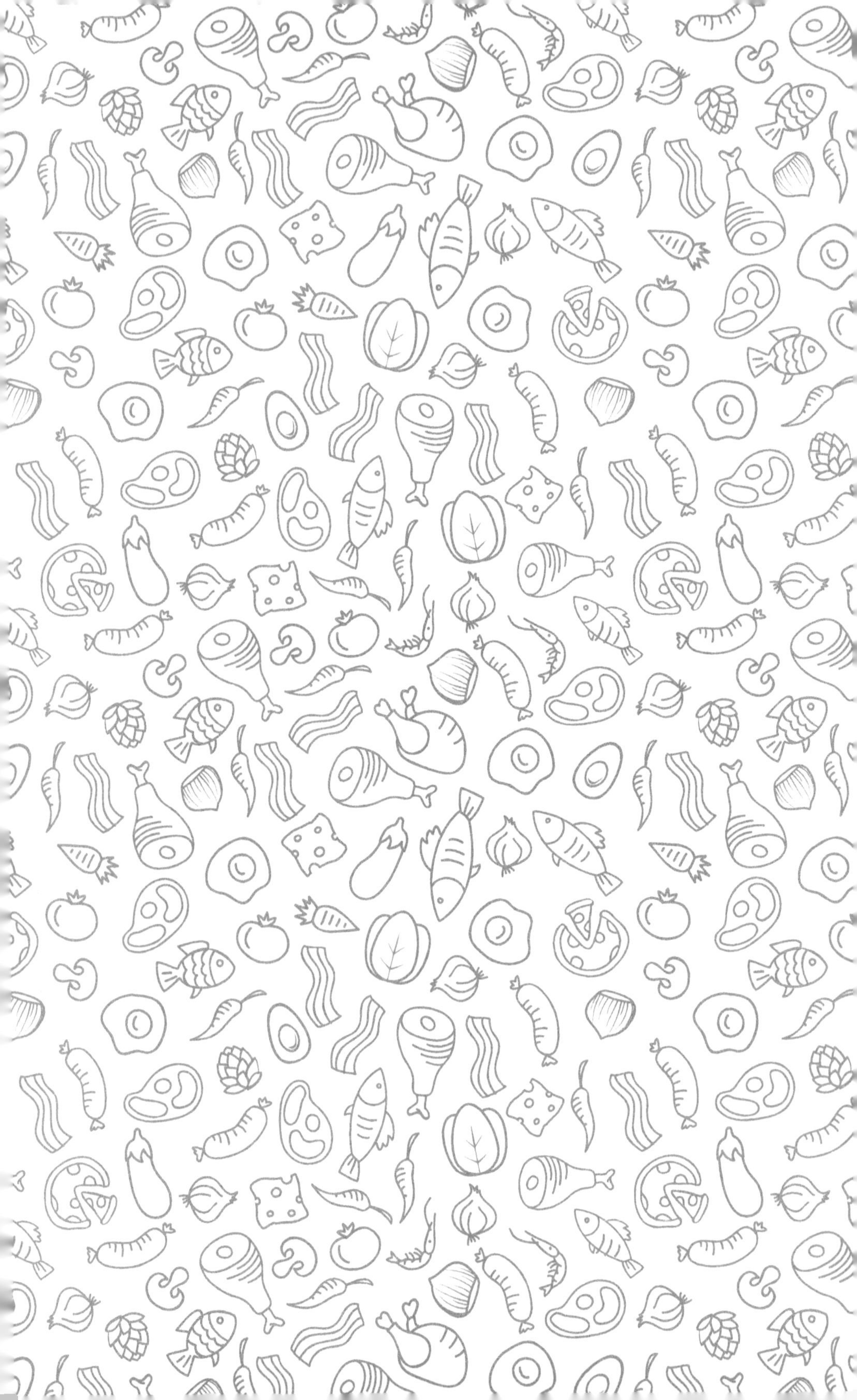

REFERENCES

[1]   U.S. Dept. of Agriculture [and] U.S. Dept. of Health and Human Services, Nutrition and your health : dietary guidelines for Americans. 1980, Washington, D.C.: U.S. Government Printing Office. *https://health.gov/dietaryguidelines/1980.asp.*

[2]   Anthanont, P. and M.D. Jensen, Does basal metabolic rate predict weight gain? Am J Clin Nutr, 2016. 104(4): p. 959-963.

[3]   Ben-Dor, M., et al., Man the Fat Hunter: The Demise of Homo erectus and the Emergence of a New Hominin Lineage in the Middle Pleistocene (ca. 400 kyr) Levant. PLOS ONE, 2011. 6(12): p. e28689.

[4]   Keys, A., Atherosclerosis: a problem in newer public health. J Mt Sinai Hosp N Y, 1953. 20(2): p. 118-39.

[5]   Keys, A., Seven countries : a multivariate analysis of death and coronary heart disease. 1980, Cambridge, Mass: Harvard University Press.

[6]   Laland, K.N., J. Odling-Smee, and S. Myles, How culture shaped the human genome: bringing genetics and the human sciences together. Nat Rev Genet, 2010. 11(2): p. 137-48.

[7]   Olalde, I., et al., Derived Immune and Ancestral Pigmentation Alleles in a 7,000-Year-old Mesolithic European. Nature, 2014. 507(7491): p. 225-228.

[8]   Eaton, S.B. and M. Konner, Paleolithic nutrition. A consideration of its nature and current implications. N Engl J Med, 1985. 312(5): p. 283-9.

[9]   Banting, W., Letter on corpulence addressed to the public. 1863: Second edition with addenda. London : Harrison and Son, 1863. *https://archive.org/details/9213279.nlm.nih.gov*

[10] Sawyer, L. and E.A. Gale, Diet, delusion and diabetes. Diabetologia, 2009. 52(1): p. 1-7.

[11] World Health Organization, Adherence to long-term therapies: evidence for action. 2003, Geneva: World Health Organization. *http://www.who.int/chp/knowledge/publications/adherence_report/en/.*

[12] Makris, A. and G.D. Foster, Dietary approaches to the treatment of obesity. Psychiatr Clin North Am, 2011. 34(4): p. 813-27.

[13] Veldhorst, M.A., M.S. Westerterp-Plantenga, and K.R. Westerterp, Gluconeogenesis and energy expenditure after a high-protein, carbohydrate-free diet. Am J Clin Nutr, 2009. 90(3): p. 519-26.

[14] Paoli, A., et al., Ketosis, ketogenic diet and food intake control: a complex relationship. Front Psychol, 2015. 6: p. 27.

[15] Merra, G., et al., Very-low-calorie ketogenic diet with aminoacid supplement versus very low restricted-calorie diet for preserving muscle mass during weight loss: a pilot double-blind study. Eur Rev Med Pharmacol Sci, 2016. 20(12): p. 2613-21.

[16] Castaldo, G., et al., An observational study of sequential protein-sparing, very low-calorie ketogenic diet (Oloproteic diet) and hypocaloric Mediterranean-like diet for the treatment of obesity. Int J Food Sci Nutr, 2016. 67(6): p. 696-706.

[17] Castaldo, G., et al., Aggressive nutritional strategy in morbid obesity in clinical practice: Safety, feasibility, and effects on metabolic and haemodynamic risk factors. Obes Res Clin Pract, 2016. 10(2): p. 169-77.

[18] de Luis, D., et al., Effect of DHA supplementation in a very low-calorie ketogenic diet in the treatment of obesity: a randomized clinical trial. Endocrine, 2016. 54(1): p. 111-122.

[19] Moreno, B., et al., Comparison of a very low-calorie-ketogenic diet with a standard low-calorie diet in the treatment of obesity. Endocrine, 2014. 47(3): p. 793-805.

[20] Bueno, N.B., et al., Very-low-carbohydrate ketogenic diet v. low-fat diet for long-term weight loss: a meta-analysis of randomised controlled trials. The British Journal of Nutrition, 2013. 110(7): p. 1178-87.

[21] Boden, G., et al., Effect of a low-carbohydrate diet on appetite, blood glucose levels, and insulin resistance in obese patients with type 2 diabetes. Ann Intern Med, 2005. 142(6): p. 403-11.

[22] Nielsen, J.V., et al., Low carbohydrate diet in type 1 diabetes, long-term improvement and adherence: A clinical audit. Diabetol Metab Syndr, 2012. 4(1): p. 23.

[23] Noakes, M., et al., Comparison of isocaloric very low carbohydrate/high saturated fat and high carbohydrate/low saturated fat diets on body composition and cardiovascular risk. Nutr Metab (Lond), 2006. 3: p. 7.

[24] Volek, J.S., et al., Carbohydrate restriction has a more favorable impact on the metabolic syndrome than a low fat diet. Lipids, 2009. 44(4): p. 297-309.

[25] Partsalaki, I., A. Karvela, and B.E. Spiliotis, Metabolic impact of a ketogenic diet compared to a hypocaloric diet in obese children and adolescents. J Pediatr Endocrinol Metab, 2012. 25(7-8): p. 697-704.

[26] Feinman, R.D., et al., Dietary carbohydrate restriction as the first approach in diabetes management: Critical review and evidence base. Nutrition, 2015. 31(1): p. 1-13.

[27] Blythman, J., Does pasta make you fat? Eight food myths busted The Guardian, 9 January 2016, [cited 15 August 2016], *https:// www.theguardian.com/lifeandstyle/2016/jan/09/does-pasta-make-you-fat-eight-food-myths-busted.*

[28] Pimpin, L., et al., Is Butter Back? A Systematic Review and Meta-Analysis of Butter Consumption and Risk of Cardiovascular Disease, Diabetes, and Total Mortality. PLoS One, 2016. 11(6): p. e0158118.

[29] Dyson, P.A., Saturated fat and Type 2 diabetes: where do we stand? Diabet Med, 2016. 33(10): p. 1312-4.

[30] Efsa Panel on Dietetic Products, N. and Allergies, Scientific Opinion on the substantiation of a health claim related to water and reduced risk of development of dehydration and of concomitant decrease of performance pursuant to Article 14 of Regulation (EC) No 1924/2006. EFSA Journal, 2011. 9(2): p. 1982-n/a.

[31] Westman, E.C., et al., Effect of 6-month adherence to a very low carbohydrate diet program. Am J Med, 2002. 113(1): p. 30-6.

[32] Dashti, H.M., et al., Long-term effects of a ketogenic diet in obese patients. Exp Clin Cardiol, 2004. 9(3): p. 200-5.

[33] Ruth, M.R., et al., Consuming a hypocaloric high fat low carbohydrate diet for 12 weeks lowers C-reactive protein, and raises serum adiponectin and high density lipoprotein-cholesterol in obese subjects. Metabolism, 2013. 62(12): p. 1779-87.

[34] Blesso, C.N., et al., Whole egg consumption improves lipoprotein profiles and insulin sensitivity to a greater extent than yolk-free egg substitute in individuals with metabolic syndrome. Metabolism, 2013. 62(3): p. 400-10.

[35] de Souza, R.J., et al., Intake of saturated and trans unsaturated fatty acids and risk of all cause mortality, cardiovascular disease, and type 2 diabetes: systematic review and meta-analysis of observational studies. Bmj, 2015. 351: p. h3978.

[36] McClellan, W.S. and E.F. Du Bois, Clinical calorimetry XLV: Prolonged meat diets with a study of kidney function and ketosis. Journal of Biological Chemistry, 1930. 87(3): p. 651-668.

[37] Volek, J.S., et al., Metabolic characteristics of keto-adapted ultra-endurance runners. Metabolism, 2016. 65(3): p. 100-10.

[38] Suez, J., et al., Non-caloric artificial sweeteners and the microbiome: findings and challenges. Gut Microbes, 2015. 6(2): p. 149-55.

[39] Suez, J., et al., Artificial sweeteners induce glucose intolerance by altering the gut microbiota. Nature, 2014. 514(7521): p. 181-6.

[40] Volek, J.S., et al., The art and science of low carbohydrate living : an expert guide to making the life-saving benefits of carbohydrate restriction sustainable and enjoyable. 2011, Lexington, KY: Beyond Obesity.

[41] Teicholz, N., The big fat surprise : why butter, meat, and cheese belong in a healthy diet. 2015.

[42] Taubes, G., The case against sugar. 2017.

[43] Oliver, E.J., Fat politics : the real story behind america's obesity epidemic. 2006, New York: University Press.

[44] Levinovitz, A., The gluten lie : and other myths about what you eat. 2015.

[45] Taubes, G., Good calories, bad calories : fats, carbs, and the controversial science of diet and health. 2008, New York: Anchor Books.

[46] Enig, M.G., Know your fats : the complete primer for understanding the nutrition of fats, oils and cholesterol. 2010, Silver Spring, MD: Bethesda Press.

[47] Eenfeldt, A. and V. Lindback, Low carb, high fat food revolution : advice and recipes to improve your health and reduce your weight. 2017.

[48] Harari, Y.N., Sapiens : a brief history of humankind. 2014: London : Harvill Secker, 2014. *https://search.library.wisc.edu/catalog/9910210845802121*.

[49] Taubes, G., Why we get fat and what to do about it. 2013.

[50] LCHFlove.com: *http://www.lchflove.com/*

[51] LCHFlove's FaceBook page: *https://www.facebook.com/LCHFlove/*

[52] Charlie Foundation: *http://www.charliefoundation.org*

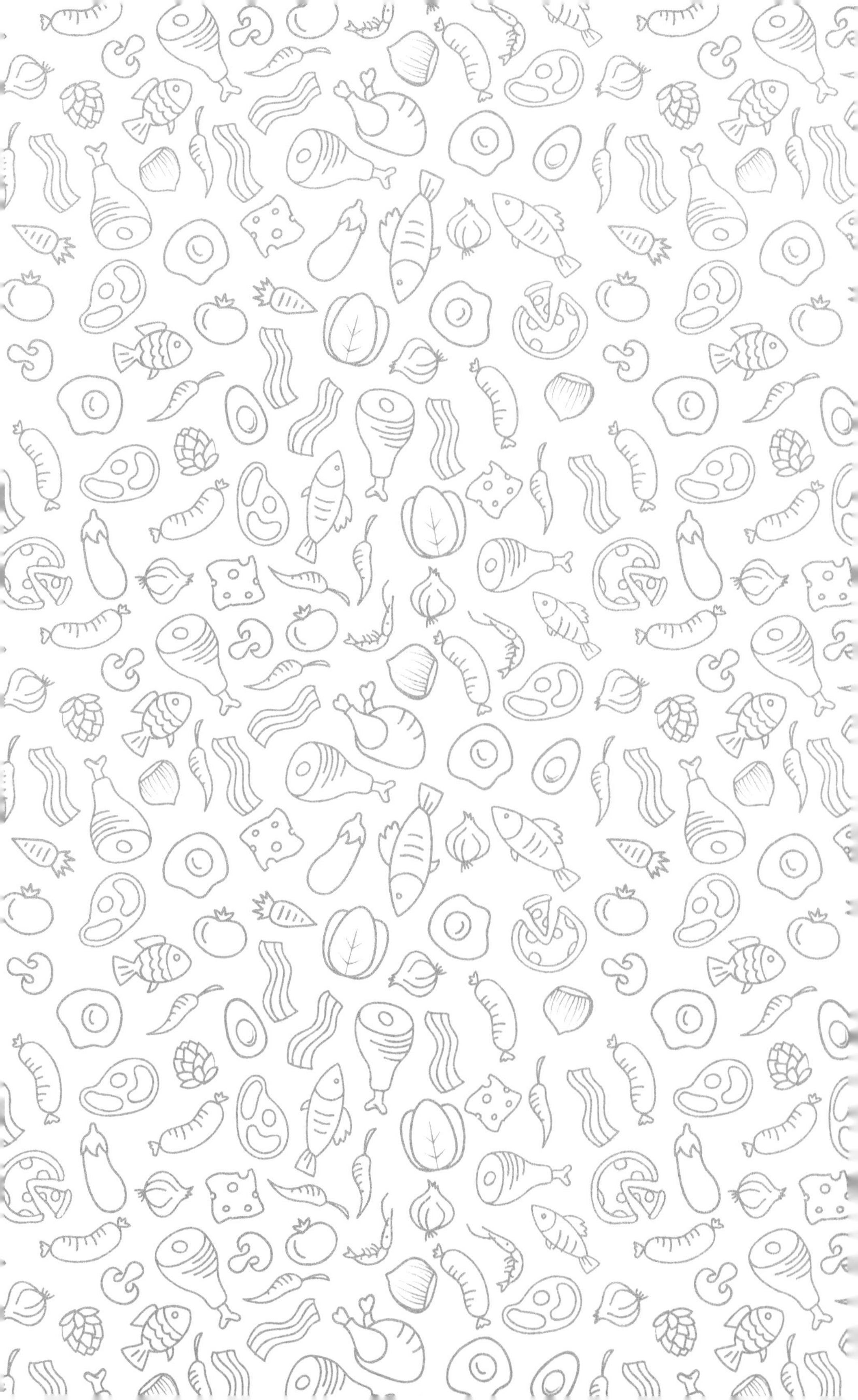

www.ingramcontent.com/pod-product-compliance
Lightning Source LLC
Chambersburg PA
CBHW051304250726
48656CB00004B/1471